CHEMISTRY RESEARCH SUMMARI1

VOLUME 12

CHEMISTRY RESEARCH SUMMARIES

Additional books in this series can be found on Nova's website under the Series tab.

Additional e-books in this series can be found on Nova's website under the e-book tab.

CHEMISTRY RESEARCH SUMMARIES

VOLUME 12

LUCILLE MONACO CACIOPPO
EDITOR

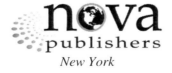

publishers
New York

For permission to use material from this book please contact us:
Telephone 631-231-7269; Fax 631-231-8175
Web Site: http://www.novapublishers.com

NOTICE TO THE READER

The Publisher has taken reasonable care in the preparation of this book, but makes no expressed or implied warranty of any kind and assumes no responsibility for any errors or omissions. No liability is assumed for incidental or consequential damages in connection with or arising out of information contained in this book. The Publisher shall not be liable for any special, consequential, or exemplary damages resulting, in whole or in part, from the readers' use of, or reliance upon, this material. Any parts of this book based on government reports are so indicated and copyright is claimed for those parts to the extent applicable to compilations of such works.

Independent verification should be sought for any data, advice or recommendations contained in this book. In addition, no responsibility is assumed by the publisher for any injury and/or damage to persons or property arising from any methods, products, instructions, ideas or otherwise contained in this publication.

This publication is designed to provide accurate and authoritative information with regard to the subject matter covered herein. It is sold with the clear understanding that the Publisher is not engaged in rendering legal or any other professional services. If legal or any other expert assistance is required, the services of a competent person should be sought. FROM A DECLARATION OF PARTICIPANTS JOINTLY ADOPTED BY A COMMITTEE OF THE AMERICAN BAR ASSOCIATION AND A COMMITTEE OF PUBLISHERS.

Additional color graphics may be available in the e-book version of this book.

Library of Congress Cataloging-in-Publication Data

ISBN: 978-1-61668-757-1
ISSN: 2327-3291

Published by Nova Science Publishers, Inc. † New York

CONTENTS

PREFACE

This new book compiles research summaries from top professionals in the field of chemistry with a number of different focuses in this important field.

In: Chemistry Research Summaries Volume 12
Editor: Lucille Monaco Cacioppo

ISBN: 978-1-61668-757-1
© 2014 Nova Science Publishers, Inc.

Chapter 1

NOVEL SYNTHETIC APPROACHES TO ION-EXCHANGEABLE METAL HYDROXIDES

Gareth Williams

School of Human Sciences, Faculty of Life Sciences,
London Metropolitan University, London, UK

RESEARCH SUMMARY

In recent years, there have been significant advances in the synthesis of hydroxides. This has led both to increased control over the composition and morphology of known hydroxides, and the development of new materials. Novel coprecipitation and hydrothermal approaches have permitted layered double hydroxides (LDHs) to be synthesised with very narrow and precisely controlled particle sizes, and have led to the synthesis of a new family of LDHs with the unprecedented stoichiometry $[MAl_4(OH)_{12}](NO_3)_2 \cdot yH_2O$ (M = Co, Ni, Cu, Zn). The use of mixed aqueous/surfactant phases during synthesis has allowed the nanosizing of LDH particles, and the production of new particle morphologies. Pioneering work by a number of researchers has led to the production of LDH thin films, with numerous potential applications. Beyond this, a range of inventive synthetic approaches have led to the discovery of myriad new hydroxide phases, including a wealth of f-block hydroxides such as the $Ln_2(OH)_5X \cdot 1.5H_2O$ (X = Cl, Br; Ln ; Y = Dy, Er, Yb) family of materials. Perhaps the culmination of this work is the recently reported synthesis of the first hydroxide framework with anion exchange properties. This chapter will discuss recent developments in hydroxide synthesis, focusing on the use of novel synthetic techniques to control product composition and morphology, highlighting the most interesting and promising new materials discovered, and enumerating potential applications arising from these scientific advances.

In: Chemistry Research Summaries Volume 12
Editor: Lucille Monaco Cacioppo

ISBN: 978-1-61668-757-1
© 2014 Nova Science Publishers, Inc.

Chapter 2

LAYERED DOUBLE HYDROXIDES APPLICATIONS AS SORBENTS FOR ENVIRONMENTAL REMEDIATION

Ricardo Rojas

INFIQC, Departamento de Fisicoquímica, Facultad de Ciencias Químicas,
Universidad Nacional de Córdoba, Ciudad Universitaria, Córdoba, Argentina

RESEARCH SUMMARY

The development of new techniques for pollution remediation is an area of high priority due to the increasing contamination of water and soils and the consequent risks to both human health and environmental equilibrium. The pollution causes are extremely diverse and, consequently, the chemicals object of remediation range from inorganic, (heavy metals, arseniate, chromate, cyanide, fluoride, etc.) to organic (petroleum by-products, pesticides, surfactants, among others). Different remediation procedures, involving chemical, biochemical or physicochemical technologies are employed according to the pollutant and the characteristics of the polluted media. One of the most widely studied is the removal or immobilization of the contaminant using sorbents such as active carbon, zeolites, ion exchange resins and layered double hydroxides (LDHs).

LDHs are mineral and synthetic compounds formed by brucite ($Mg(OH)_2$)-like layers with partial isomorphic substitution by trivalent cations. This replacement leads to a positive charge excess compensated by anions weakly bonded by electrostatic forces and placed in the interlayer space. LDHs present an huge customization capacity: a wide range of metal ions, either divalent (Mg^{2+}, Ca^{2+}, Ni^{2+}, Fe^{2+}, Zn^{2+}, Cd^{2+}, Cu^{2+},...) or trivalent (Al^{3+}, Fe^{3+}, Cr^{3+},...) can be arranged in the layers. Different anions (from simple and small inorganic anions such as chloride, nitrate or carbonate, to large organic and biological anions such as surfactants, pharmaceutical drugs, and even biomolecules) can also be included due to these solids capacity to expand the interlayer distance.

The main features of these solids are a high anion exchange capacity (around 3 meq/g), the layers instability at low pHs and the capacity to reconstruct its lamellar structure from the oxides obtained by their calcination. Due to their anion exchange properties, LDHs are studied as sorbents for a wide variety of water pollutants either inorganic (arseniate, chromate) or organic (pesticides, dyes) anions. The contaminant uptake during the reconstruction process of calcined LDHs has also been extensively studied and the acid base buffering properties of LDHs produce heavy metal ions precipitation as hydroxides, either as part of the hydroxylated layers or in a separate hydroxide phase. Also, due to their customization capacity, the environmental applications of LDHs can be extended: modification of LDHs with organic anions allows adsorption of neutral or even positively charged apolar species in the interlayer or in the surface of the solids and the intercalation of polydentate ligands such as citrate, malate and ethylenediaminetraacetate (EDTA) modifies the metal ions uptake capacity of the hydroxylated layers. In this chapter, the LDHs properties will be described and their uptake mechanisms analyzed. On this base, their applications as pollutant scavengers will be reviewed and analyzed, highlighting the factors that affect the sorbents behavior and the customization strategies used to obtain an optimal performance.

In: Chemistry Research Summaries Volume 12   ISBN: 978-1-61668-757-1
Editor: Lucille Monaco Cacioppo   © 2014 Nova Science Publishers, Inc.

Chapter 3

UTILITY OF SODIUM AND POTASSIUM HYDROXIDES FOR PREPARING SUPERIOR QUALITY ACTIVATED CARBONS

A. Linares-Solano, M. A. Lillo-Ródenas, J. P. Marco-Lozar, M. Kunowsky and A. J. Romero-Anaya*

Dpto. Química Inorgánica, Universidad de Alicante, Spain

RESEARCH SUMMARY

Alkaline hydroxides, especially sodium and potassium hydroxides, are multi-million-ton per annum commodities and strong chemical bases that have large scale applications. Some of them are related with their consequent ability to degrade most materials, depending on the temperature used. As an example, these chemicals are involved in the manufacture of pulp and paper, textiles, biodiesels, soaps and detergents, acid gases removal (e.g., SO_2) and others, as well as in many organic synthesis processes. Sodium and potassium hydroxides are strong and corrosive bases, but they are also very stable chemicals that can melt without decomposition, NaOH at 318°C, and KOH at 360°C. Hence, they can react with most materials, even with relatively inert ones such as carbon materials. Thus, at temperatures higher than 360°C these melted hydroxides easily react with most types of carbon-containing raw materials (coals, lignocellulosic materials, pitches, etc.), as well as with most pure carbon materials (carbon fibers, carbon nanofibers and carbon nanotubes). This reaction occurs via a solid-liquid redox reaction in which both hydroxides (NaOH or KOH) are converted to the following main products: hydrogen, alkaline metals and alkaline carbonates, as a result of the carbon precursor oxidation. By controlling this reaction, and after a suitable washing process, good quality activated carbons (ACs), a classical type of porous materials, can be prepared.

Such carbon activation by hydroxides, known since long time ago, continues to be under research due to the unique properties of the resulting activated carbons. They have promising high porosity developments and interesting pore size distributions. These two properties are

---

* Corresponding Author. Fax; +34 965903454. E-mail address: linares@ua.es (A. Linares-Solano).

important for new applications such as gas storage (e.g., natural gas or hydrogen), capture, storage and transport of carbon dioxide, electricity storage demands (EDLC-supercapacitors-) or pollution control. Because these applications require new and superior quality activated carbons, there is no doubt that among the different existing activating processes, the one based on the chemical reaction between the carbon precursor and the alkaline hydroxide (NaOH or KOH) gives the best activation results.

The present chapter covers different aspects of the activation by hydroxides, including the characteristics of the resulting activated carbons and their performance in some applications. The following topics are discussed: i) variables of the preparation method, such as the nature of the hydroxide, the type of carbon precursor, the hydroxide/carbon precursor ratio, the mixing procedure of carbon precursor and hydroxide (impregnation of the precursor with a hydroxide solution or mixing both, hydroxide and carbon precursor, as solids), or the temperature and time of the reaction are discussed, analyzing their effect on the resulting porosity; ii) analysis of the main reactions occurring during the activation process, iii) comparative analysis of the porosity development obtained from different activation processes (e.g., CO_2, steam, phosphoric acid and hydroxides activation); and iv) performance of the prepared activated carbon materials on a few applications, such as VOC removal, electricity and gas storages.

In: Chemistry Research Summaries Volume 12
Editor: Lucille Monaco Cacioppo

ISBN: 978-1-61668-757-1
© 2014 Nova Science Publishers, Inc.

Chapter 4

Delamination of Layered Double Hydroxides: Methodologies, Characterization and Applications

Churchil A. Antonyraj, Paulmanickam Koilraj and Kannan Srinivasan[*]

Discipline of Inorganic Materials and Catalysis,
Central Salt and Marine Chemicals Research Institute,
Council of Scientific and Industrial Research (CSIR), GB Marg, India

Research Summary

Layered double hydroxides (LDHs) are ionic lamellar compounds that consist of positively charged metal hydroxide sheets and interlayers filled with anions. They are expressed by the general formula $[M^{2+}_{(1-x)}M^{3+}_x(OH)_2]A^{n-}_{x/n}.mH_2O$, wherein M^{2+} and M^{3+} are any divalent and trivalent metal ions capable of occupying the octahedral vacancies of brucite-like sheets and A^{n-} is any hydrated anion. The act of slicing or peeling of laminated layers into individual layers or sheets is called delamination and is also referred as exfoliation. Due to high charge density of the layers that result in strong electrostatic interaction, delamination of LDHs remained a challenge. Pioneering work by Prof. Besse and coworkers broke that then prevailing ideology to delaminate layers of LDHs in organic medium. LDHs on delamination give nanosheets of thickness around 1–5 nm with several micron in lateral dimensions and possess novel physical and chemical properties, compare to their corresponding microcrystalline powder form. Recently, the delaminated materials showed potential applications in films for sensing, composites for packaging, selective removal of noxious anions in trace concentrations, functional coatings, erasable high density information storage, electrochemical applications, anti-reflection coatings, optoelectronics and catalysis. In this chapter, we review the delamination of LDHs including the genesis, different methodologies adopted in the last decade, characterization of delaminated

[*] Tel: +91-278-2567760 Ext. 703; Fax: +91-278-2567562; E-mail: skannan@csmcri.org ; kanhem1@yahoo.com.

nanosheets and their applications in diverse domains. A novel and scalable two-step synthesis protocol of transition metal containing delaminated LDHs in water as dispersing medium developed in our laboratory and their characterization are presented. Different strategies employed in delaminating LDHs with an endeavor to obtain high degree of delamination are discussed. An ingenious first time exploration of using delaminated LDHs for phosphate removal in environmental perspective is highlighted. Mechanism of phosphate uptake by delaminated LDHs is unraveled. A model pond system is conceptualized for onsite phosphate remediation and demonstrated on laboratory scale. The scope and further utilization of delaminated LDHs is summarized.

In: Chemistry Research Summaries Volume 12
Editor: Lucille Monaco Cacioppo
ISBN: 978-1-61668-757-1
© 2014 Nova Science Publishers, Inc.

Chapter 5

α–PHASE LAYERED HYDROXIDES, SYNTHESIS, TYPES, NANOHYBRIDS

Mohammad Yeganeh Ghotbi
Ceramic Engineering Department, Faculty of Engineering,
Malayer University, Malayer, Iran

RESEARCH SUMMARY

The α–phase metal hydroxides are layered materials whose structure is similar to that of the better studied layered hydroxides, LDHs. They also have positively charged layers formed solely with divalent cations within brucite-like sheets. These layered hydroxides are important materials owing to their ability to intercalate or ion-exchange various functional anions. This leads to the production of the materials with new physico-chemical properties for use in diverse technological areas. Moreover, αLHs and their nanohybrids have been suitable precursors to make undoped and doped nanostructured metal oxides, metal and metal alloys as well as carbon materials and metal oxide carbon composites.

In: Chemistry Research Summaries Volume 12
Editor: Lucille Monaco Cacioppo

ISBN: 978-1-61668-757-1
© 2014 Nova Science Publishers, Inc.

Chapter 6

ANIONIC DEPOLLUTION BY LAYERED HYDROXIDES

F. Delorme[1,*] and A. Seron[2]

[1]GREMAN, CNRS-CEA, Université François Rabelais,
BLOIS, France
[2]BRGM, ORLEANS Cedex, France

RESEARCH SUMMARY

Human activities have generated numerous pollutions due to heavy metals. Therefore, many remediation processes have been developed to trap these cations. Moreover, materials presenting cation-exchange properties such as clays are very common.

Pollutions due to anions have been less studied in the past even if they can be of major importance in some areas, due to geological aspects and/or human activities. The utmost critical and studied anionic pollution, which is a major public health problem, is certainly the presence of arsenic in drinking waters of Bangladesh. Indeed, the average As concentration in water in Bangladesh is 0.06 mg.l^{-1}, with values as high as 16 mg.l^{-1}. These values are far beyond the 0.01 mg.l^{-1} threshold fixed by the World Health Organization. However, many other anions can be the cause of various pollution. Human activities can generate important concentrations of fluoride in water. Tanzania is one of the most affected countries: indeed, concentrations in piped waters as high as 8 mg.l^{-1} during the rainy season and 12.7 mg.l^{-1} during the dry season are observed. The threshold value fixed by the World Health Organization values is 1.5 mg.l^{-1}, far below the concentrations observed in Tanzania. Intensive agricultural activities are known to generate nitrates water pollutions. This is the case of Brittany, the western part of France, where nitrates concentrations up to 250 mg.l^{-1} can be observed. These values are far beyond the 50 mg.l^{-1} WHO threshold. And many other similar examples concerning chromates, phosphates, selenium, chlorides, vanadates, sulfates, molybdates, mercury chlorides or cyanides could be mentioned.

Nowadays no pertinent and economical depollution processes are useful for such applications : most of them are complicated to use (biological ones) or generate big amounts

---

*Corresponding author: Tel.: +33-2-54-55-21-10; Fax: +33-2-54-55-21-37; E-mail: fabiandelorme@yahoo.fr.

of by-products (zerovalent iron). Nevertheless innovative solutions could be furnished using materials with anionic exchange capacity.

Unfortunately, materials presenting anion-exchange properties are less abundant than materials presenting cation-exchange properties. The main family of materials presenting anion-exchange properties are layered hydroxides. Two different families of layered hydroxides are mainly studied: Layered Double Hydroxides ($[M(II)_{1-x}M(III)_x(OH)_2]$ $[A^{n-}]_{x/n} \cdot mH_2O$) containing both divalent and trivalent cations, and Double Hydroxide Salts that only contains divalent cations.

The synthesis and structure of these materials will be presented in this chapter, as well as the origin of their anion exchange properties and their potential for anionic depollution.

In: Chemistry Research Summaries Volume 12   ISBN: 978-1-61668-757-1
Editor: Lucille Monaco Cacioppo   © 2014 Nova Science Publishers, Inc.

Chapter 7

CERAMIC PIGMENTS FROM MIXED HYDROXIDES WITH THE HYDROTALCITE-LIKE STRUCTURE

V. Rives[1,*], M. E. Pérez-Bernal[1], R. J. Ruano-Casero[1] and I. Nebot-Díaz[2]

[1]GIR-QUESCAT, Departamento de Química Inorgánica,
Universidad de Salamanca, Spain
[2]Escola Superior de Cerámica de L'Alcora, Castellón, Spain

RESEARCH SUMMARY

The preparation, characterisation and structural properties of layered double hydroxides with the hydrotalcite-like structure are described, as well as those of solids formed upon their thermal decomposition in air. Characterisation of these hydroxides by powder X-ray diffraction, Fourier Transform Infrared (FT-IR) spectroscopy, electron microscopy, thermal methods (thermogravimetric and differential thermal analyses) is described.

The most widely preparation methods used (namely, coprecipitation, salt-oxide method, urea hydrolysis, sol-gel, etc.) and post-synthesis treatments (ageing and hydrothermal treatment, both under conventional or microwave heating) are described and discussed.

The different factors controlling the properties of these hydroxides and those of the solids formed upon their thermal decomposition and their use as ceramic pigments are discussed. The method of preparation and the nature of the mixed hydroxides used provide a unique method for preparation of pigments with almost any pursued colour.

---

* Corresponding author: Professor Vicente Rives, address as above. Tel.: +34 923 29 44 89; Fax: :34 923 29 45 74;
  E-mail: vrives@usal.es.

In: Chemistry Research Summaries Volume 12
Editor: Lucille Monaco Cacioppo

ISBN: 978-1-61668-757-1
© 2014 Nova Science Publishers, Inc.

Chapter 8

SYNTHESIS, CHARACTERISATION AND APPLICATIONS OF GENUINE LAYERED DOUBLE HYDROXIDE THIN FILMS

Mónika Sipiczki[1], Pál Sipos[1] and István Pálinkó[2]

[1]Department of Inorganic and Analytical Chemistry, University of Szeged, Hungary
[2]Department of Organic Chemistry, University of Szeged, Hungary

RESEARCH SUMMARY

The synthesis and characterisation of various L(ayered)D(ouble)H(ydroxide) thin film types are overviewed here, together with applications. Those substances are only considered that keep their layered structure in the form of thin film *and* in the case of composite structures LDHs play the role of the host. Methods of preparation and structural features are discussed for the pure LDH, the inorganic-inorganic as well as organic-inorganic host-guest complex films. Optical and conductive properties of the films are displayed together with any other important properties with an emphasis on applications as sensors of various kinds.

In: Chemistry Research Summaries Volume 12   ISBN: 978-1-61668-757-1
Editor: Lucille Monaco Cacioppo   © 2014 Nova Science Publishers, Inc.

Chapter 9

CHARACTERIZATION OF LAYERED DOUBLE HYDROXIDES BY NEAR INFRARED SPECTROSCOPY

César Jiménez-Sanchidrián and José Rafael Ruiz[*]

Departamento de Química Orgánica, Facultad de Ciencias,
Universidad de Córdoba, Campus de Rabanales, Córdoba, Spain

RESEARCH SUMMARY

This paper reviews the results of recent studies on the characterization of layered double hydroxides (LDHs) by near infrared spectroscopy (NIRS). The properties of LDHs containing various cations and interlayer anions are discussed. Basically, NIRS allows the nature of OH groups present in LDHs to be established and bands due to electronic transitions in LDHs containing metals with *d* orbitals to be identified.

[*] E-mail: qo1ruarj@uco.es.

In: Chemistry Research Summaries Volume 12 ISBN: 978-1-61668-757-1
Editor: Lucille Monaco Cacioppo © 2014 Nova Science Publishers, Inc.

Chapter 10

PREPARATION AND CHARACTERIZATION OF IN(OH)₃: EU NANOSTRUCTURES OBTAINED BY MICROWAVE-ASSISTED HYDROTHERMAL METHOD

Fabiana V. Motta[1,*], Ana Paula A. Marques[2], Carlos A. Paskocimas[1], Mauricio R. D. Bomio[1], Maria Fernanda C. Abreu[3], Máximo S. Li[4], Edson R. Leite[3], José A. Varela[5] and Elson Longo[5]

[1]Laboratório de Síntese Química, Departamento de Engenharia de Materiais, Universidade Federal do Rio Grande do Norte, Natal, RN, Brazil
[2]Departamento de Ciências Exatas e da Terra, Universidade Federal de São Paulo, Diadema, SP, Brazil
[3]Laboratório Interdisciplinar de Eletroquímica e Cerâmica, Departamento de Química, Universidade Federal de São Carlos, São Carlos, SP, Brazil
[4]Instituto de Física de São Carlos, Universidade de São Paulo, São Carlos, SP, Brazil
[5]Laboratório Interdisciplinar de Eletroquímica e Cerâmica, Instituto de Química, Universidade Estadual Paulista, Araraquara, SP, Brazil

RESEARCH SUMMARY

Crystalline europium-doped indium hydroxide (In(OH)₃:Eu) nanostructures were prepared by a rapid and efficient Microwave-Assisted Hydrothermal (MAH) method. Nanostructures were obtained at a low temperature. FE-SEM images confirm that these samples are composed of 3D nanostructures. XRD, optical diffuse reflectance and photoluminescence (PL) measurements were used to characterize the products. Emission spectra of europium-doped indium hydroxide samples under excitation (350.7 nm) presented broad band emission referent to the indium hydroxide (In(OH)₃) matrix and $^5D_0 \rightarrow {}^7F_0$, $^5D_0 \rightarrow {}^7F_1$, $^5D_0 \rightarrow {}^7F_2$, $^5D_0 \rightarrow {}^7F_3$ and $^5D_0 \rightarrow {}^7F_4$ europium transitions at 582, 596, 618, 653 and 701 nm, respectively. Relative intensities of the Eu^{3+} emissions increased as the concentration of this ion increased from 0, 1, 2, 4 and 8 mol %, of Eu^{3+}, but the luminescence is drastically quenched for the In(OH)₃ matrix.

In: Chemistry Research Summaries Volume 12 ISBN: 978-1-61668-757-1
Editor: Lucille Monaco Cacioppo © 2014 Nova Science Publishers, Inc.

Chapter 11

APPLICATION OF SOLID HYDROGEN PEROXIDE FOR TOOTH WHITENING THERAPY

*Morimichi Mizuno**

School of Dentistry, Hokkaido University, Sapporo, Japan

RESEARCH SUMMARY

Hydrogen peroxide has been widely used by dentists for vital tooth whitening to improve the esthetics of the dentition during two decade. Now two types of whitening therapy are practiced, one is in-office whitening using hydrogen peroxide gel, and the other is home whitening using carbamide peroxide gel. Though these procedures are accepted for tooth whitening, there are several serious problems in management and stability of hydrogen peroxide. These problems are basically owing to fluidity of the reagent. To resolve these problems, I developed a new technology to solidify hydrogen peroxide solution.

Solid hydrogen peroxide (Shp) has following features.

1. Shp is easy for handling and has no irritant activity for skin and mucous membrane when keeping dry condition.
2. Shp is stable for a longer time than hydrogen peroxide solution. Shp keeps bleaching activity at least one month at room temperature; on the other hand, same amount of hydrogen peroxide solution loses activity within 5 days by the evaporation.
3. Shp is able to immortalize on synthetic resin. It is possible to form the hybrid resin containing hydrogen peroxide.
4. Shp fixes easily and tightly on tooth surface compared with commercial whitening reagent.

Shp was applied for vital tooth whitening, and was recognized that more than 90% of patients felt the effect of therapy within one week.

---

* Mail address: mmizuno@den.hokudai.ac.jp (mizunom0923@yahoo.co.jp).

Therefore, Shp is superior to commercial whitening reagent as regarding effect and management.

In: Chemistry Research Summaries Volume 12
Editor: Lucille Monaco Cacioppo

ISBN: 978-1-61668-757-1
© 2014 Nova Science Publishers, Inc.

Chapter 12

REACTIVITY OF PORPHYRIN RADICAL CATIONS AND DICATIONS TOWARDS NUCLEOPHILES: AN EASY AND ORIGINAL ELECTROCHEMICAL METHOD FOR THE SYNTHESIS OF SUBSTITUTED, OLIGOMERIC AND POLYMERIC PORPHYRIN SYSTEMS

Delphine Schaming[1], Alain Giraudeau[2] and Laurent Ruhlmann[1,2]

[1] Laboratoire de Chimie Physique,
Université Paris-Sud (Paris 11), Orsay, France
[2] Laboratoire d'Electrochimie et de Chimie-Physique
du Corps Solide, Université de Strasbourg, Strasbourg, France

RESEARCH SUMMARY

The electrochemical properties of porphyrins are now well established. Indeed, it is well known that the oxidation of the π-ring of a porphyrin proceeds *via* two one-electron steps generating the π-radical cation and the dication. The reactivity of porphyrin π-radical cations and dications with nucleophilic compounds has also been intensively studied. For instance, a direct electrochemical oxidation of the β-octaethylporphyrin (OEP) in the presence of pyridine as Lewis base leads to substitutions of protons by pyridiniums in *meso*-positions onto the macrocycle. Mechanism of such *meso*-substitutions is based on nucleophilic attacks of the Lewis bases onto the electrooxidized macrocycle and is described as an ECEC process. Similarly, such an electrochemical oxidation of the *meso*-tetraphenylporphyrin (TPP) leads to β-substitutions by pyridiniums. A similar reactivity of the oxidized porphyrins has also been observed in using phosphanes as nucleophilic groups instead of pyridyl groups.

Furthermore, this method has allowed the electrosynthesis of dimers, and more generally oligomers, of porphyrins, either in using 4,4'-bipyridine which possesses two nucleophilic sites, or in using porphyrins substituted by pendant pyridyl group(s). The control of the degree of substitution of the oligomers obtained is permitted by a judicious choice of the applied potential or in varying the number of pyridyl groups onto the porphyrin used as Lewis base, respectively. Then, dimers and oligomers obtained possess pyridinium or viologen spacers having interesting electrochemical properties.

Moreover, this reactivity-type of porphyrins has also allowed the development of an original and easy methodology for the electropolymerization of porphyrins, in using porphyrins and species having two nucleophilic sites. Such electropolymerization is performed with iterative scans by cyclic voltammetry. With this method of electropolymerization, it is possible to modulate easily the nature of the bridging spacers between the porphyrin macrocycles, allowing the formation of polymers with specific chemical and structural properties. Moreover, this novel way of electropolymerization opens up also interesting synthesis routes for the elaboration of new functional materials. Indeed, for instance, copolymers containing two different types of porphyrins can be obtained in using porphyrins substituted by pendant pyridyl groups. Original organic-inorganic copolymers can also be obtained in using inorganic compounds functionalized by two pendant pyridyl groups. For example, inorganic compounds such as polyoxometalates, having interesting catalytic properties, can be employed, the presence of the porphyrin within the copolymer allowing then a photosensibilization for applications in photocatalysis.

In: Chemistry Research Summaries Volume 12   ISBN: 978-1-61668-757-1
Editor: Lucille Monaco Cacioppo   © 2014 Nova Science Publishers, Inc.

Chapter 13

MAKING PORPHYRINS TO FEEL LIKE AT HOME

*M. A. García-Sánchez[*1], F. Rojas González[1], S. R. Tello Solís[1], E. C. Menchaca Campos[2], I. Y. Quiroz Segoviano[1], V. de la Luz[1], L. A. Díaz Alejo[1], E. Salas Bañales[1] and A. Campero[1]*

[1] Department of Chemistry, Universidad Autónoma
Metropolitana-Iztapalapa, México
[2] Centro de Investigación en Ingeniería y Ciencias Aplicadas,
UAEM, Morelos, México

RESEARCH SUMMARY

The important physicochemical and technological properties displayed by free porphyrins in solution have been preserved or even enhanced through the disaggregated physical or chemical trapping of these species inside solid networks (e.g., SiO_2, ZrO_2, TiO_2, etc.) synthesized by the sol-gel technique. The physical trapping of porphyrins or phthalocyanines can be performed inside SiO_2 networks; nevertheless, the interaction of encapsulated macrocyclic species with silanol (Si-OH) groups attached to the pore walls can promote the aggregation or degradation of these molecules thus inhibiting their inherent fluorescent or catalytic properties.

These deleterious effects can be overcome by exchanging the -SiOH surface groups by *alkyl* groups ensuing from organo-substituted alkoxides. The presence of these *alkyl* groups changes the polarity inside the pores, even though this strategy not always precludes ill effects over the optical and luminescent properties of the trapped macrocyclic species. A second alternative consists in chemically bonding porphyrins to the pore walls through bridges created from the reaction between functionalized alkoxides and organic substituting groups located at the periphery of the porphyrin molecule. Through this methodology, translucent and monolithic xerogels have been obtained although the fluorescence properties of the porphyrins fixed to the pore walls are just partially preserved. The average pore cavity diameters in which the macrocyclic species can be located range from 2.1 to 3.6 nm.

---

[*] Tel. 58044677, e-mail: mags@xanum.uam.mx

Nevertheless, a third option consists in binding substituted porphyrinic species to the pore walls through large chemical bridges created from the combination between functionalized alkoxides and polymer precursors, such as diamines, diacids or lactams. As a result of this exploration, monomeric or oligomeric porphyrins can also be trapped inside SiO_2 networks.

These oligomeric species can be formed from the reaction between tetraphenylporphyrins functionalized with –COOH or –NH_2 groups and the polymer precursors mentioned above. By following this methodology the fluorescence properties of porphyrins bonded to the pore walls of translucent and monolithic silica networks result similar to those shown by the free macrocyclic species in solution.

The characterization analysis reveals the creation of pore sizes ranging from 4.4 to 9.4 nm, which could only be possible if more than one porphyrin molecule is trapped inside the pore. By reason of the above properties, these new hybrid solids systems can be successfully applied in catalytic, sensing, optical, and medical devices. The covalent bonding of porphyrins to the pore walls of organo-modified silica matrices is the most recent strategy that is being explored by our research group for modeling the solid chemical environment in which porphyrins can be trapped while displaying their original luminescent properties similar to those found in solution.

In: Chemistry Research Summaries Volume 12
Editor: Lucille Monaco Cacioppo

ISBN: 978-1-61668-757-1
© 2014 Nova Science Publishers, Inc.

Chapter 14

SYNTHETIC STRATEGIES TO CHLORINS AND BACTERIOCHLORINS

Marta Pineiro, Arménio C. Serra
and Teresa M. V. D. Pinho e Melo
Department of Chemistry, University of Coimbra, Coimbra, Portugal

RESEARCH SUMMARY

Chorin and bacteriochlorin molecules (hydroporphyrins) are the ones chosen by Nature to interact with light whether in direct light capture or in subsequent electronic transfer processes. The reason lies in the fact that these molecules present high absortion capacity in the red and near-infrared region and also easy oxidation-reduction reactions. The possibility of introducing metals in these molecules and the modulation of physical properties by changing the structural periphery are also important characteristics. In our search for artificial system to get closer to the natural ones it is very important to have tools to assist in the preparation of these classes of macrocycles. This review provides an updated overview of the more relevant contributions to the synthesis of chlorins and bacteriochlorins. Chlorins and bacteriochlorins have been prepared via pericyclic reactions namely Diels-Alder reactions, 1,3-dipolar cycloadditions, [$8\pi+2\pi$] cycloadditions and cheletropic reactions. Synthetic approaches to hydroporphyrins also involve the reduction and oxidation of porphyrins as well as nucleophilic and electrophilic addition to porphyrins. The more relevant methodologies for the total synthesis of chlorins and bacteriochlorins from pyrrole derived precursors are also discussed.

In: Chemistry Research Summaries Volume 12   ISBN: 978-1-61668-757-1
Editor: Lucille Monaco Cacioppo   © 2014 Nova Science Publishers, Inc.

Chapter 15

RECENT ACHIEVEMENTS FOR CHEMICAL SENSING, TUMOR MARKER DETECTION AND CANCER THERAPY WITH PORPHYRIN DERIVATIVES

Kamil Záruba[1], Pavel Řezanka[1], Pavel Žvátora[1],
Zdeněk Kejík[1,2], Pavel Martásek[2] and Vladimír Král[1,3]

[1]Institute of Chemical Technology Prague, Prague, Czech Republic
[2] First Faculty of Medicine, Charles University in Prague,
Prague, Czech Republic
[3]Zentiva Development, Part of Sanofi Group, Prague, Czech Republic

RESEARCH SUMMARY

Porphyrins represent an interesting family of compounds with a broad field of applications. From all of them, we have focused on those based on their strong interaction with light. High molar absorptivity and high quantum yield of fluorescence due to their unique electronic structure based on a cyclic array of adjacent π orbitals are precursors for applications of porphyrins in analytical sensing development and medicinal therapy based on interaction of a tissue with light. The broad field of the use of porphyrins forces us to divide the chapter into several parts.

The most recent achievements in porphyrin synthesis are briefly summarized at the beginning. Part two is devoted to applications in analytical chemistry mainly based on porphyrin spectrochemical sensors development (primarily absorption and fluorescence sensors). Herein, porphyrin derivatives have been utilized in solution and at the gas-solid and/or liquid-solid interfaces. The final part of the review deals with cancer therapy using porphyrins. The approach leading to selective destruction of tumor cells is called photodynamic therapy (PDT) and porphyrins act here as so called photosensitizers. Beside a short general survey of PDT with porphyrins and others photosensitizers, the last development of porphyrin photosensitizers based on their enhanced tumor cells targeting is reviewed.

In: Chemistry Research Summaries Volume 12
Editor: Lucille Monaco Cacioppo

ISBN: 978-1-61668-757-1
© 2014 Nova Science Publishers, Inc.

Chapter 16

USE OF THE PORPHYRIN AUTOFLUORESCENCE FOR CANCER DIAGNOSIS

Lilia Coronato Courrol[1],
Flavia Rodrigues de Oliveira Silva[2]
and Maria Helena Bellini[3]*

[1]Departamento de Ciências Exatas e da Terra,
Universidade Federal de São Paulo, Diadema, SP –Brazil
[2] Centro de Ciência e Tecnologia de Materiais, IPEN/CNEN-SP, São Paulo, SP –Brazil
[3]Centro de Biotecnologia, IPEN/CNEN-SP, São Paulo, SP –Brazil

RESEARCH SUMMARY

The diagnosis of premalignant lesions is of great importance because it increases the chances of cure and prevention of the high risk of tumor spread to other organs (metastasis). δ-Aminolevulinic acid (ALA) is a precursor of porphyrin in the heme biosynthesis pathway.

When an excessive amount of exogenous ALA is given, one of the intermediated products of heme-cycle, the protoporphyrin IX (PpIX), accumulates in the cells. PpIX is an oncotropic photosensitiser that provides an intense red fluorescence when blue light at a wavelength around 400 nm is used. ALA-induced PpIX has been used for photodynamic diagnosis (PDD) or photodynamic therapy (PDT) to identify or kill tumor cells allowing cancer diagnosis and therapy. In this review, the mechanism of PpIX accumulation in tumor cells, and the potential of ALA-induced PDD in situ or for blood samples are discussed. Furthermore, the animal model of primary prostate cancer is used to describe and to analyze the application of ALA-induced PpIX fluorescence as a tumor marker.

---

* Email: lccourrol@gmail.com

In: Chemistry Research Summaries Volume 12   ISBN: 978-1-61668-757-1
Editor: Lucille Monaco Cacioppo   © 2014 Nova Science Publishers, Inc.

Chapter 17

PORPHYRINS: CHEMISTRY, PROPERTIES AND APPLICATIONS

Tien Quang Nguyen, Mary Clare Sison Escaño and Hideaki Kasai[*]

Department of Applied Physics, Graduate School of Engineering,
Osaka University, Osaka, Japan

RESEARCH SUMMARY

During the past decade, porphyrin and its derivatives have been widely studied due to their numerous physical/chemical properties and their applications in many fields such as catalysis, sensors and photodynamic cancer therapy, among others. A porphyrin molecule is a heterocyclic macrocycle derived from four pyrroline subunits interconnected through their α-carbon atoms and methine bridges (=CH-). The porphyrin molecule can coordinate hydrogen or metal cations in its center by four isoindole nitrogen atoms. The structural, electronic and magnetic properties of porphyrin can be well modified by varying the metal at its center or adding ligands onto the organic rings, making them attractive candidates for many applications. Metal porphyrins have been considered as one of the potential cathode catalysts for Polymer Electrolyte Fuel Cells (PEFCs), where the oxygen reduction reaction (ORR) takes place. In nature, this reaction to oxygen can be modeled by iron-porphyrin (FeP) - a part of heme considered as active site of enzymes such as hemoglobin, which transports O_2 molecules in vascular systems and cytochrome oxidase where O_2 is activated in an aerobic metabolism. Also, porphyrin is considered as one of the building blocks of several porphyrin complexes of different conjugation types such as *tape-porphyrin* and *sheet-porphyrin*. For instance, tape-porphyrin, whose adjacent building blocks are fully linked via two β-carbon bonds and one *meso*-carbon bond, has attracted much attention due to its extremely small highest occupied - lowest unoccupied molecular orbital (HOMO-LUMO) gap making them useful for molecular electronic devices like sensors and switches for gas detection.

[*] Tel: +81-6-6879-7857; Fax: +81-6-6879-7859; Email: kasai@dyn.ap.eng.osaka-u.ac.jp

In: Chemistry Research Summaries Volume 12　　　ISBN: 978-1-61668-757-1
Editor: Lucille Monaco Cacioppo　　　© 2014 Nova Science Publishers, Inc.

Chapter 18

APPLICATIONS OF PORPHYRINS FOR NEOANGIOGENIC DISORDERS

Sang Geon Kim, Jung Min Lee and Woo Hyung Lee

College of Pharmacy, Seoul National University, Seoul, Korea

RESEARCH SUMMARY

Porphyrins are a group of cyclic organic macromolecules composed of four modified pyrrole subunits. They are composed of tetrapyrroles backbone, metal, and side chains (e.g., propionic acid, methyl and vinyl). Binding of divalent metal cation to tetrapyrrole backbone results in the final mitochondrial synthesis of different porphyrins. As a component of hemoproteins, heme plays a role in transporting gaseous molecules in the blood, contributing to the regulation of the cardiovascular system. In fact, several porphyrins have been clinically applied to treat certain diseases; hemin has been prescribed for the treatment of porphyria attacks in acute intermittent porphyria. Protoporphyrin, another porphyrin prototype, has also been studied as a potent hepatoprotective and choleretic agent in liver disease. Recent research results have also suggested the applications of porphyrins as anti-cancer agents based on their abilities to inhibit inflammation and angiogenesis. This chapter will cover not only the chemical properties and biosynthesis of porphyrins, but also the recent reports on their applications. This information may offer insight into the use of porphyrins as therapeutic agents, especially with regard to the inhibition of neoangiogenesis, and tumor progression and proliferation.

In: Chemistry Research Summaries Volume 12   ISBN: 978-1-61668-757-1
Editor: Lucille Monaco Cacioppo   © 2014 Nova Science Publishers, Inc.

Chapter 19

MOLECULAR ENCAPSULATION OF STRUCTURALLY DIFFERENT QUINONES BY PORPHYRIN-RESORCIN [4] ARENE CONJUGATES

Talal F. Al-Azemi[*], *Mickey Vinodh and Abdirahman A. Mohamod*
Department of Chemistry, Kuwait University, Safat, Kuwait

RESEARCH SUMMARY

Calix-and resorcin[4]arene cavitands have been extensively studied in recent years because of their attractive artificial receptor characteristics and possessing multipoint recognition ability towards noncovalently bound guest molecules. Resorcin[4]arenes which are cyclic tetramers of resorcinol are synthesized in reasonably high yields via simple, one phase, and acid-catalyzed condensation reaction. Structural modification of the resorcin[4]arene macrocycle is carried out to introduce one alkyl bromide function on the structure for further chemical transformations. The hydroxyl groups of the upper resorcinarene rims are bridged together to give the rigid, bowl shaped cavitand or methylated with iodomethane to provide an open flexible conformation. Such conformational modifications enabled resorcin[4]arenes to operate as diverse and effective hosts in supramolecular chemistry for the attachment of different ligating sites giving rise to ionophores for anions, cations and neutral molecules. Combination of porphyrins which are suitable class of compounds for building artificial molecular devices because of their photoactive and electronic properties with resorcin[4]arene provides wide prospects in the design of selective receptors and supersensitive sensors. *meso*-5-(3-Hydroxyphenyl) 10,15,20-(4-toluyl)porphyrin is prepared by condensation of pyrrole and appropriate phenyl aldehydes. Porphyrin-resorcin[4]arene conjugates were synthesized by reaction of the alkyl bromide function of the resorcinarene unit with hydroxy function of the porphyrins. Proper molecular design enabled the porphyrin-resorcin[4]arene coupling to occur where the porphyrin core is preferably oriented above the resorcin[4]arene cavity to make these systems suitable for molecular encapsulation and selective catalysis. The influence of the

[*] Corresponding author: Tel.: +965-2498-5540; fax: +965-2481-6482; e-mail: t.alazemi@ku.edu.kw

resorcin[4]arene fragment on the porphyrin fluorescence was investigated by using four structurally different quinones –benzoquinone (BQ), 1,4-naphthoquinone (NQ), phenanthrenequinone (PAQ) and dichlorodicyanobenzoquinone (DDQ). The data shows that at low concentration of quinone, the fluorescence quenching of the porphyrin considerably enhanced by the attachment of resorcin[4]arene to the photoactive subunit which is supported by ^{1}H NMR experiments. These types of conjugates present interesting opportunities for various applications such as artificial enzyme mimics.

In: Chemistry Research Summaries Volume 12
Editor: Lucille Monaco Cacioppo

ISBN: 978-1-61668-757-1
© 2014 Nova Science Publishers, Inc.

Chapter 20

PORPHYRIN SOLID FILMS: GROWING PROCESSES, PHYSICAL FEATURES, AND OPTICAL PROPERTIES

Michele Tonezzer[1,2,3]

[1]Dipartimento di Ingegneria dei Materiali e Tecnologie Industriali,
Università di Trento, Trento, Italy
[2]Legnaro National Laboratories – INFN, Legnaro (PD), Italy
[3]LEITAT Technological Center - Terrassa, Barcelona, Spain

RESEARCH SUMMARY

Porphyrins are widespread compounds in nature, where they play essential functions for life. The porphyrin molecule contains four pyrrole rings linked via methine bridges (see Figure 1) and porphyrin nucleus is a tetradentate ligand in which the space available for a coordinated metal has a maximum diameter of approximately 3.7 A. The porphyrin ring system is stable and exhibits aromatic character: almost all metals form complexes 1:1, although Na, K, Li complexes are 2:1 in which the metal are incorporated slightly below and above the porphyrin macrocycle plane. Porphyrin metal complexes play an important role in biological activities as for instance iron complex in the haemoproteins, magnesium complexes in the chlorophylls, and a cobalt complexin Vitamin B12. Porphyrin derivatives play a key role in essential biological processes such as photosynthesis, dioxygen transport and storage.

Porphyrin ligand has turned out to be very versatile, and almost all metals have been combined with porphyrins. Such complexes have been used in a variety of applications as models for biologicalelectron transport, oxygen transport and metalloenzymes. It is well known that porphyrin is also a highsensitive chromogenic reagent owing to the fact that porphyrins andtheir metal chelates generally exhibit characteristicsharp and intensive absorption bands in the visibleregion. Thanks to its photochemical and redox activity, the porphyrinmacrocycle is an attractive building block on which to append additional recognition sites for anion binding.

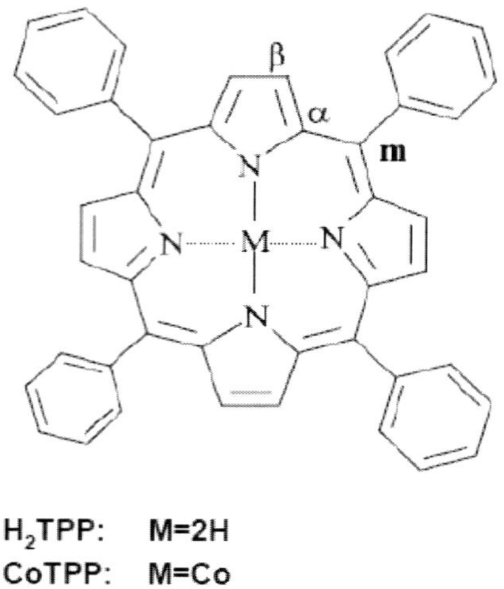

H$_2$TPP: M=2H
CoTPP: M=Co

Figure 1. Structure of metal free (H$_2$TPP) and cobalt (CoTPP) meso-tetra phenyl porphyrin and atom labelling scheme.

In: Chemistry Research Summaries Volume 12
Editor: Lucille Monaco Cacioppo

ISBN: 978-1-61668-757-1
© 2014 Nova Science Publishers, Inc.

Chapter 21

ELECTROCATALYTIC REDUCTION OF OXYGEN BY COBALT PORPHYRINS FOR FUEL CELL APPLICATIONS

Shawn Swavey

Department of Chemistry, University of Dayton, Dayton, Ohio, US

RESEARCH SUMMARY

With the ever-present need to move away from a dependence on foreign oil, scientists need the tools to develop alternative energy sources, including fuel cells and, more specifically, new and better cathode catalysts for fuel cells. Many advances in cathode catalysis development have taken place over the past three decades however a replacement for platinum, a costly and easily poisoned catalyst, has yet to be realized. Cobalt porphyrins catalyze oxygen reduction very near the potential reached by platinum catalysts and they are typically less expensive. Unfortunately a typical cobalt porphyrin catalyst reduces oxygen by two electrons to hydrogen peroxide instead of the more desired four electron reduction to water. In addition, the stability of cobalt porphyrins under fuel cell conditions has been an ongoing concern preventing commercialization. This chapter will discuss some of the past three decades work in the area of cobalt porphyrin catalysts including some of the very interesting ways researchers have tried to improve their stability as well as enhance their catalytic ability.

In: Chemistry Research Summaries Volume 12
Editor: Lucille Monaco Cacioppo

ISBN: 978-1-61668-757-1
© 2014 Nova Science Publishers, Inc.

Chapter 22

CYCLOADDITION REACTIONS AS THE KEY STEP IN THE SYNTHESIS OF COVALENTLY LINKED PORPHYRIN-FULLERENE SUPRAMOLECULAR SYSTEMS

Davor Margetić[1]

Laboratory for Physical Organic Chemistry, Division of Organic
Chemistry and Biochemistry, Rudjer Bošković Institute,
Zagreb, Croatia

RESEARCH SUMMARY

This review describes the utilization of cycloaddition reactions in the organic synthesis of porphyrin-fullerene molecular architectures, where two functionalities are covalently linked together. Proper choice of cycloaddends was found to be crucial for efficient assembly of exceedingly complex supermolecular porphyrin-fullerene conjugates. Synthetic power of cycloaddition reactions have been recognized by researchers dealing with the areas of new photoactive organic materials as crucial components for efficient artificial light-harvesting, energy and charge transfer processes.

[1] e-mail: margetid@irb.hr.

In: Chemistry Research Summaries Volume 12
Editor: Lucille Monaco Cacioppo

ISBN: 978-1-61668-757-1
© 2014 Nova Science Publishers, Inc.

Chapter 23

PHOSPHORUS (V) PORPHYRIN: ITS POTENTIAL APPLICATION FOR PHOTOMEDICINE

Kazutaka Hirakawa
Department of Basic Engineering (Chemistry),
Faculty of Engineering, Shizuoka University, Japan

RESEARCH SUMMARY

Porphyrin derivatives are used as photosensitizers for photodynamic therapy, which is a less invasive cancer phototherapy. The mechanism of photodynamic therapy is the biomacromolecule's damage through a photosensitized reaction. Singlet oxygen, which is formed through the energy transfer to molecular oxygen from the photoexcited porphyrins, causes the oxidation of biomacromolecules, such as protein and/or DNA, during photo-irradiation. On the other hand, photo-induced electron transfer is also an alternative mechanism of photodynamic therapy. High-valent porphyrin complexes, including phosphorus(V)porphyrins, demonstrate a lower redox potential of one-electron reduction in their photoexcited state than free base or low-valent metal complexes. Therefore, these porphyrins are advantageous for oxidative electron transfer reactions. Phosphorus(V)porphyrins can photosensitize the damage of DNA and protein through dual mechanisms of singlet oxygen generation and electron transfer. These porphyrins have the potential as a novel photosensitizer to attack cancer cells under the low-oxygen environment of a tumor through the electron transfer.

In: Chemistry Research Summaries Volume 12
Editor: Lucille Monaco Cacioppo

ISBN: 978-1-61668-757-1
© 2014 Nova Science Publishers, Inc.

Chapter 24

CONSTRUCTION AND SUPRAMOLECULAR CHEMISTRY OF PORPHYRIN NANORINGS

*Akiharu Satake**

Department of Chemistry, Faculty of Science, Tokyo University of Science,
Shinjuku-ku, Tokyo, Japan

RESEARCH SUMMARY

Light-harvesting antenna complexes (LH-I and LH-II) in photosynthetic purple bacteria are naturally occurring porphyrin-derivative nanorings. This review focuses on the construction and supramolecular chemistry of artificial porphyrin nanorings, where the porphyrins are located closely and interact strongly with one another, in a similar manner to LH-I and LH-II. In particular, three unique systems, *meso–meso* directly linked porphyrins, butadiyne-linked porphyrins, and imidazole-to-zinc complementary coordinating porphyrins are reviewed in detail.

---

* E-mail: satake@rs.kagu.tus.ac.jp.

In: Chemistry Research Summaries Volume 12   ISBN: 978-1-61668-757-1
Editor: Lucille Monaco Cacioppo   © 2014 Nova Science Publishers, Inc.

Chapter 25

PORPHYRINS: PROPERTIES AND APPLICATIONS

Whittney N. Burda[1], Lindsey N. Shaw[1] and Mark Shepherd[2]

[1]Department of Cell Biology, Microbiology and Molecular Biology,
University of South Florida, Tampa, Florida, US
[2]School of Biosciences, University of Kent, Canterbury, UK

RESEARCH SUMMARY

Porphyrins are organic molecules consisting of four pyrrole rings connected via their α-carbon atoms by methine (=CH-) bridges. Although not all porphyrins share the same optical properties, the name for 'porphyrin' comes from the Greek name for purple, which eludes to the striking colour elicited by an intricate connectivity of carbon atoms: the extensive network of alternating (conjugated) double bonds and resultant delocalised π-electron cloud that shrouds the porphyrin macrocycle gives rise to the intense optical absorbance and fluorescent properties. Most biological porphyrins are able to coordinate metal ions, yielding metalled-porphyrins required for a vast range of biological processes, including light harvesting in photosynthesis, electron transport in respiration, and oxygen transport in the blood. While biological porphyrins are crucial for a variety of cellular processes, an accumulation of porphyrins in the presence of light and oxygen can be highly toxic to living cells: porphyrins may absorb light energy resulting in an excited quantum state that can react with molecular oxygen to produce reactive oxygen species such as singlet oxygen and superoxide. It is this property of porphyrins that makes them suitable for the treatment of cancer by photodynamic therapy, where synthetic porphyrins are targeted to the site of the tumour followed by irradiation with a laser. Similar approaches are currently under development for porphyrin antimicrobials, which may provide the next line of defence against microorganisms that have evolved resistance to multiple antibiotics. The chemical properties of metallated porphyrins have also been exploited for the destruction of tumor cells in cancer patients. Hence, porphyrins are crucial for life on earth, and have important clinical applications.

In: Chemistry Research Summaries Volume 12
Editor: Lucille Monaco Cacioppo

ISBN: 978-1-61668-757-1
© 2014 Nova Science Publishers, Inc.

Chapter 26

CHALLENGES AND PERSPECTIVES OF IONIC LIQUIDS VS. TRADITIONAL SOLVENTS FOR CELLULOSE PROCESSING

John Gräsvik[1], Dilip G. Raut[1] and Jyri-Pekka Mikkola[1,2]
[1]Technical Chemistry, Department of Chemistry,
Chemical-Biological Center, Umeå University, Umeå, Sweden
[2]Industrial Chemistry and Reaction Engineering, Process Chemistry Centre,
Åbo Akademi University, Åbo-Turku, Finland

RESEARCH SUMMARY

It is commonly accepted that world-wide production of oil, coal and natural gas will eventually come to a halt, although we still heavily depend on these non-renewable feed stocks and their associated chemical derivatives. Therefore, new, sustainable resources for the production of industrially important chemicals are required. Biomaterials offer much promise in this regard, since they generally contain a lot of cellulose which can be transformed and potentially provide a great source of industrially important chemicals. Presently, only a small part of the annual biomass growth in the world is utilized by industry, while the rest is decaying along natural pathways. In order to effectively process cellulose, it needs to be dissolved in some liquid medium. Present state-of-the-art commercial technologies employ very toxic and hazardous processing with volatile organic solvents like CS_2. However, this need not be the case. Ionic liquids (ILs) have shown great potential for the dissolution of cellulose. Some ILs also have attractive physical properties such as: low vapor pressure, high thermal stability and reusability. Thus, they are potentially viable and more environmentally friendly alternatives. Hereby, we present and discuss some of the challenges and perspectives for ILs in terms of their potential for cellulose processing. We briefly review the historical processes and current methods for cellulose processing, and look at alternative processes taking advantage of ILs.

In: Chemistry Research Summaries Volume 12
Editor: Lucille Monaco Cacioppo

ISBN: 978-1-61668-757-1
© 2014 Nova Science Publishers, Inc.

Chapter 27

IONIC LIQUIDS AS SUSTAINABLE EXTRACTANTS IN PETROCHEMICALS PROCESSING

G. Wytze Meindersma, Antje R. Hansmeier, Ferdy S. A. F. Onink and André B. de Haan*
Eindhoven University of Technology,
Dept. of Chem. Eng and Chem./SPS, The Netherlands

RESEARCH SUMMARY

Only a few ionic liquids can be successfully applied for the separation of aromatic hydrocarbons from mixtures of aromatic and aliphatic hydrocarbons. Ionic liquids have been identified as promising solvents to replace conventional solvents in liquid-liquid extraction of aromatic hydrocarbons requiring less process steps and less energy consumption, provided that the mass-based aromatic distribution coefficient and/or the aromatic/aliphatic selectivity are higher than those of the current state-of-the-art solvents such as sulfolane. The most suitable ionic liquids from our evaluation are [3-mebupy]B(CN)$_4$, [3-mebupy]C(CN)$_3$, [3-mebupy]N(CN)$_2$ and [bmim]C(CN)3. The aromatic distribution coefficients of these ILs are a factor of 1.2 to 2.5 higher and the aromatic/aliphatic selectivities are up to a factor of 1.9 higher than with sulfolane.

A process evaluation of the extraction of aromatic hydrocarbons with ionic liquids shows that a high aromatic distribution coefficient with a reasonable aromatic/aliphatic selectivity could reduce the investment costs of the aromatic/aliphatic separation by a factor of two compared to a conventional separation with e.g., sulfolane.

The separation of aromatic and aliphatic hydrocarbons from complex streams with multiple aromatics, e.g., naphtha, is one of the central separation steps within oil refineries. The evaluation of real feeds in comparison to model feeds is essential in order to study the extraction behaviour of ionic liquids with highly complex feed mixtures and, therewith, to evaluate the suitability of ionic liquids for industrial aromatic extraction processes. Although

---

* Email: g.w.meindersma@tue.nl

the amount is less for real refinery streams than for the investigated model feeds, a good separation is obtained.

Ionic liquids can also extract mono- and poly-aromatic sulfur and nitrogen components from gasoline and diesel fuels. Since these compounds are responsible for the formation of smog, sour gases, acid rain and NO_x emissions, these heterocyclic components have to be removed. From all refinery streams contributing to the gasoline blending pool, FCC gasoline is with up to 2.5 wt.% sulfur content the main sulfur source in carburant fuels. In order to meet the current compulsory limits for the sulfur content in carburant fuels, i.e., gasoline (petrol) and diesel fuels, the sulfur content has to be reduced to 10 ppm.

The ionic liquids [3-mebupy]$N(CN)_2$, [4-mebupy]$N(CN)_2$, [4-mebupy]SCN and [bmim]$C(CN)_3$ are superior for sulfur removal compared to sulfolane which has been used as benchmark. These ionic liquids exhibit an up to 20% higher capacity in case of thiophene and in the case of dibenzothiophene even up to 53%. Furthermore, it has been shown that nitrogen containing hetero-aromatic components are significantly better extracted than sulfur components.

The results from laboratory equilibrium experiments for both the extraction of aromatics from mixtures of aromatic and aliphatic hydrocarbons and the removal of sulfur and nitrogen compounds from fuels have been validated with [4-mebupy]BF_4 (aromatic removal) and [3-mebupy]$N(CN)_2$ and sulfolane (removal of both aromatics and S- and N-compounds) in our 6 m high pilot plant extraction column. The ionic liquid [3-mebupy]$N(CN)_2$ has been found to be the best ionic liquid in terms of mass based capacity and can outperform sulfolane for the removal of aromatic hydrocarbons and for the removal of sulfur and nitrogen containing components from both model and real refinery streams.

In: Chemistry Research Summaries Volume 12   ISBN: 978-1-61668-757-1
Editor: Lucille Monaco Cacioppo   © 2014 Nova Science Publishers, Inc.

Chapter 28

IONIC LIQUIDS IN ELECTROANALYTICAL CHEMISTRY: A REVIEW FOR THE FURTHER DEVELOPMENT AND APPLICATIONS

*Weena Siangproh[1], Wijittar Duangchai[2] and Orawon Chailapakul[3,4]**

[1]Department of Chemistry, Faculty of Science,
Srinakharinwirot University, Bangkok, Thailand
[2]Department of Chemistry, Faculty of Science,
King Mongkut's University of Technology Thonburi,
Bangkok, Thailand
[3]Department of Chemistry, Faculty of Science, Chulalongkorn University,
Bangkok, Thailand
[4]National Center for Excellence Petroleum,
Petrochemicals and Advanced Materials, Chulalongkorn University,
Patumwan, Bangkok, Thailand

RESEARCH SUMMARY

Nowadays, the scientific and technological importance of ionic liquids (ILs) have expanded a wide range of applications, owing to their unique physicochemical properties, such as thermal and chemical stability, low melting point, negligible volatility, flame retardancy, high ionic conductivity, moderate viscosity, high polarity, and solubility /affinity with many compounds. Electrochemical processes have been another important application area for ILs. The advantages of ILs over common aqueous or organic media in this field are their wide electrochemical window, high conductivity, and vanishingly low vapor pressure. The most important advances in this field depend on the development of new sensors for various applications. This chapter will discussed of the properties of ILs and their general applications based on these properties, especially the application of ILs in electroanalytical

* Corresponding author: Orawon Chailapakul E-mail: corawon@chula.ac.th Tel and Fax: +662-218-7615

area. They concerned the current achievements and their applicability in electroanalytical measurements within the period of 2006-2011.

In: Chemistry Research Summaries Volume 12
Editor: Lucille Monaco Cacioppo

ISBN: 978-1-61668-757-1
© 2014 Nova Science Publishers, Inc.

Chapter 29

BRÖNSTED ACID-BASE IONIC LIQUIDS AND MEMBRANES AS ION CONDUCTING MATERIALS: SYNTHESIS, PROPERTIES AND APPLICATIONS

Harinder Pal Singh Missan and Marisa Singh*

Fuel Cell Materials Research Lab, Department of Physics,
University of West Indies, St. Augustine, Trinidad and Tobago, WI

RESEARCH SUMMARY

Ionic liquids (IL's) are salts in which the ions are poorly coordinated, resulting in these solvents being liquid below $100^{\circ}C$, or even at room temperature (room temperature ionic liquids, RTIL's). They are nonflammable, have low vapor pressure, high ionic conductivity and excellent chemical and thermal stability over a large temperature range. IL's can be synthesized in a wide range of structures and many IL's have even been developed for specific applications and processes. One such group of IL's is Brönsted acid - base IL's. This system operates such that the Brönsted base functions as an acceptor of protons of the Brönsted acids and thus creates a Grotthuss mechanism based proton conduction path in the ionic liquids. One of the applications of Brönsted acid – base IL's which are used in various morphologies and configurations includes membranes for fuel cells, the simplest approach being a supported liquid membrane. Other applications for Brönsted acid – base IL's include sensors, electrochemical capacitor, electrochromic windows etc. IL's can also be used as a liquid in a membrane contactor, where the liquid viscosity is an important factor which can be controlled by changing temperature and they can be functionalized to incorporate unsaturated carbon–carbon bonds that can be used to form polymers. Recent morphology advancement is the formation of gelled structures has improved mechanical properties in comparison to the liquid while still retaining the diffusion properties of a liquid phase. Since the solubility characteristics remain very similar to the liquid, the resulting permeability when used as a membrane is very similar to a liquid membrane but with improved mechanical properties.

---

* Corresponding author. Email: harinder.missan@sta.uwi.edu, Phone: 1-868-662-2002 Extn. 3116 (off.), 1-868-662-9904 (Fax), 1-868-479-0945 (Cell)

IL's have been shown to provide benefits in composite structures containing two or more components that are combined to obtain a performance that is not possible with just one component. There are various methods to synthesize these structures. One approach is to incorporate IL's into the polymer. Thus, the material will maintain the solubility selectivity while enhancing the diffusion rate across the membrane since the material now has a more "liquid-like" behaviour. The IL is contained in the membrane due to the strong electrostatic interactions with both the liquid and the ionic polymer. Also, a three component mixed matrix membrane has been developed that alleviates the problem associated with the lack of adhesion between the membrane and the solid phase. Ionic liquid is added to the material that wets both the polymer and the solid. This wetting phase provides a selective layer between the solid and polymer. Since the IL is nonvolatile, it remains in the membrane. IL's are therefore leaving their mark in the development of membranes for fuel cell applications. In this review, different Brönsted acid - base IL systems and membranes based on them has been discussed to determine their suitability and applicability for fuel cells.

In: Chemistry Research Summaries Volume 12
Editor: Lucille Monaco Cacioppo

ISBN: 978-1-61668-757-1
© 2014 Nova Science Publishers, Inc.

Chapter 30

THE PHYSICAL AND CHEMICAL PROPERTIES OF IONIC LIQUIDS AND ITS APPLICATION IN EXTRACTION

Yu Cao, Shun Yao, Xiaoming Wang,
Qi Peng and Hang Song[*]
Department of Pharmaceutical and Biological Engineering,
Sichuan University, Chengdu, China

RESEARCH SUMMARY

Ionic liquids (ILs) as green solvents are attracting increasing interest from industry and academic in the whole world during past years. The researches on ILs are developing at an incredible rate. Their negligible vapor pressure, high thermal stability and relatively high viscosity make them different from the conventional organic solvents. This review focuses on the major physical and chemical properties of ILs related to the extraction application including polarity, pH value, melting point and solubility, etc. The review take some examples to illustrate the applications of ILs in various subjects of extraction, including extraction of biological molecular, active components from natural products, organic compounds from other resources except natural products and metal ions, etc. Current status of the application of ILs in the extraction and most significant achievements were reviewed. The comparison between traditional organic solvents and ILs in the application of extraction suggested that ILs would be a potential excellent solvent with wide application range in various extraction processes.

[*] corresponding author: hangsong@vip.sina.com

In: Chemistry Research Summaries Volume 12
Editor: Lucille Monaco Cacioppo

Chapter 31

THE USE OF IONIC LIQUIDS FOR DYE-SENSITIZED SOLAR CELLS

*Chuan-Pei Lee[1] and Kuo-Chuan Ho[1,2]**
[1]Department of Chemical Engineering, and
[2]Institute of Polymer Science and Engineering
National Taiwan University, Taipei, Taiwan

RESEARCH SUMMARY

This chapter mainly deals with the topic of ionic liquids (ILs) for the use as the electrolyte in dye-sensitized solar cells (DSSCs). A brief review on five strategies of using ILs for improving the performance or durability in DSSCs will be introduced. Firstly, the application of molten salts, triethylamine hydroiodide (THI) and tetraethylammonium iodide (TEAI), as supporting electrolytes were synthesized and investigated for the DSSCs. Optimum cell efficiency (η) of 8.45% were obtained for the DSSC containing 0.5 M of THI/0.05 M iodine (I_2)/0.5 M 4-tert-butylpyridine (TBP) in acetonitrile (ACN). In the second strategy, binary ILs of imidazolium salts containing different cations and anions were used as electrolytes in quasi-solid-state DSSCs, and their physicochemical properties were also studied on the cell performances. The DSSC with a binary ILs electrolyte reaches an η of 4.11% and shows a superior long-term stability. As the third strategy, gel-type DSSCs were fabricated with ILs electrolyte containing poly-1,1'-(methylenedi-4,1-phenylene) bismaleimide (PBMI) prepared by *in situ* polymerization of the corresponding monomer without an initiator at 30 °C. By adding the exfoliated alkyl-modified nanomica (EAMNM) into the gel electrolyte, the corresponding DSSC shows higher η of 7.02% than that with PBMI-gel electrolytes without EAMNM (6.41%) and this also resulted in remarkably stable cell performance under continuous light soaking of one sun at 55 °C. The fourth strategy is to fabricate a near-solid-state DSSC by using 1-propyl-3-methylimidazolium iodide (PMII) and polyaniline-loaded carbon black (PACB) as the composite electrolyte without the addition of iodine. With the addition of 1-ethyl-3-methylimidazolium thiocyanate (EMISCN, a lower

* E-mail address: kcho@ntu.edu.tw

viscosity IL), the η of 6.15% is achieved with this type of DSSC. At-rest durability of the DSSC with binary IL/PACB composite electrolyte was studied at 70 °C and shows unfailing durability. The last one is based on a solid IL crystal, 1-ethyl-3-methylimidazolium iodide (EMII), employed as a charge transfer intermediate (CTI) to fabricate an all-solid-state DSSC. In addition, single-walled carbon nanotubes (SWCNTs) were incorporated into EMII and achieved a higher η of 1.88%, as compared to that containing bare EMII (0.41%). Moreover, PMII, which acts simultaneously as a co-CTI and crystal growth inhibitor, was used to further improve η. The highest η (3.49%) is achieved using a hybrid SWCNT-binary CTI and shows a durability of greater than 1,000 h at room temperature.

In: Chemistry Research Summaries Volume 12
Editor: Lucille Monaco Cacioppo

ISBN: 978-1-61668-757-1
© 2014 Nova Science Publishers, Inc.

Chapter 32

GEMINI DICATIONIC ACIDIC IONIC LIQUIDS: SYNTHESIS, PROPERTIES AND CATALYTIC APPLICATIONS

Yingwei Zhao, Xiaofei Liu, Zhen Li, Jing Chen and Chungu Xia**

State Key Laboratory for Oxo Synthesis and Selective Oxidation,
Lanzhou Institute of Chemical Physics,
Chinese Academy of Sciences, Lanzhou, China

RESEARCH SUMMARY

The sulfonic acid ($-SO_3H$) functionalized ionic liquids have attracted much attention in the green procedure of acid-catalyzed organic reactions. Herein, we report on the synthesis and characterization of a series of novel gemini dicationic sulfonic acid-functionalized ionic liquids based on imidazole, pyrrolidine, and morpholine, respectively. The detailed studies on the physicochemical properties of these dicationic ionic liquids showed that they are thermally stable and electrochemically inert, and possess higher density and viscosity compared with common monocationic sulfonic acid-functionalized ionic liquids. They also showed noticeable hydrophilic properties and stronger acidities, which make them more efficient in catalytic reactions. The dicationic acidic ionic liquids based on pyrrolidine exhibited excellent performance in esterification, and up to 99% yield was obtained when 5 mol% of ionic liquids was used. The imidazole-based ionic liquids mediated $ZnCl_2$ are also good catalysts for Beckmann rearrangement of oximes. The morpholine-based ionic liquids could catalyze the selective alkylation of phenol with *t*-butyl alcohol and the product distribution was found related to the acidity of the catalyst. Furthermore, all these ionic liquids could be reused for several times without appreciable loss of efficiency, exhibiting good stability.

* Corresponding author: zhenli@licp.cas.cn; cgxia@licp.cas.cn

In: Chemistry Research Summaries Volume 12   ISBN: 978-1-61668-757-1
Editor: Lucille Monaco Cacioppo   © 2014 Nova Science Publishers, Inc.

Chapter 33

TASK-SPECIFIC IONIC LIQUID-CATALYZED CONVERSION OF CARBON DIOXIDE INTO FUEL ADDITIVE AND VALUE-ADDED CHEMICALS

Zhen-Zhen Yang, Ya-Nan Zhao and Liang-Nian He[*]
The State Key Laboratory and Institute of Elemento-Organic Chemistry,
Nankai University, Tianjin, P. R. China

RESEARCH SUMMARY

As an abundant, nontoxic, nonflammable, easily available, and renewable carbon resource, carbon dioxide (CO_2) is very attractive as an environmentally friendly feedstock for making commodity chemicals, fuels, and materials. Owing to its kinetic inertness and thermodynamic stability, significant efforts have been directed towards constructing C-C, C-O and C-N bond on the basis of CO_2 activation through molecular catalysis. Development of catalytic methodologies for chemical transformation of CO_2 into useful compounds is of paramount importance from a standpoint of C1 chemistry and Green. Chem.istry. In this chapter, we would like to illustrate potential applications of CO_2 in the synthesis of fuel additive/industrial useful chemicals by employing task-specific ionic liquids (TSILs) as catalysts/reaction media.

Those findings summarized herein would open synthetic pathways for the selective synthesis of heterocycles such as cyclic carbonates and oxazolidinones as well as industrial important compounds from CO_2 and demonstrate that such CO_2 functionalization with high energy starting material like epoxides is easily operative and practical in industry. We believe that CO_2 chemistry disclosed in this chapter including our recent work performed at Nankai University, will stimulate further interest in research that may lead to the development of CO_2 as a C1 building block for a wide set of value-added organic compounds like solvents, fuels, fine/bulk chemicals, pharmaceuticals and polymers.

[*] Email: heln@nankai.edu.cn.

In: Chemistry Research Summaries Volume 12   ISBN: 978-1-61668-757-1
Editor: Lucille Monaco Cacioppo   © 2014 Nova Science Publishers, Inc.

Chapter 34

IONIC LIQUIDS AND SMART SEPARATIONS TECHNOLOGY FOR METAL REMOVAL FROM WASTEWATERS

F. J. Alguacil, I. Garcia-Diaz, F. A. Lopez, O. Rodriguez, A. Urien and I. Padilla*

Centro Nacional de Investigaciones Metalurgicas (CSIC), Madrid, Spain

RESEARCH SUMMARY

Properties of ionic liquids make these compounds of interest in a wide number of applications. Due to their composition, a cation and an anion, these compounds can be used also advantageously in separation processes.

Pollution of the environment is one of the problems to be solved by mankind. Many metals are considered as hazardous elements and thus their removal from wastewaters are needed to protect the environment and to avoid poisoning of animal species and humans. Despite their toxicity, metals and their compounds found a wide variety of uses in agriculture, industry and medicine.

In this chapter, recent applications of ionic liquids and three separations technology are considered. The coupling of both ionic liquids and separations technology can be used to improve the removal of metals from wastewaters before its final disposal or convenient recycling or even yielding a saleable product.

Liquid-liquid extraction is a proven technology for the recovery of heavy metals and is useful in medium and large scale operations and when the solute concentration is high. In the operation, the ionic liquid, sometimes dissolved in a suitable diluent, is contacted with the waste stream and the metal or solute transfers into the organic phase. This loaded organic phase is then further contacted with a second or strip aqueous phase. The extracted species transfer back into the strip phase, from which is finally processed and also the organic phase is regenerated and is returned to a further extraction process.

---

* Corresponding author E-mail: fjalgua@cenim.csic.es

Liquid membranes technologies using organic phases extended the range of conditions under which liquid-liquid extraction processes are viable. The organic phases used in these technologies resembled very closely to those used in liquid-liquid extraction operation. The term liquid membrane is given to a system in which the membrane that divides the feed and stripping phases consists of a thin film or organic solution. In supported liquid membranes (SLMs) the organic phase is immobilized in the pores of a porous polymer. The polymeric support, which is generally of hydrophobic nature, consists of microporous membranes in the form of a sheet or hollow fiber. The polymer is wet by the organic solution, which filled the pores to produce the liquid membrane. This then forms a physical barrier between the aqueous feed and strip solutions. Recent and smart modifications to SLMs operation mode, in which ionic liquids are used as carrier phase, include: polymer-inclusion liquid membranes (PILMs), pseudo-emulsion membrane strip dispersion (PEMSD), and pseudo-emulsion hollow fiber strip dispersion (PEHFSD).

Ion-exchange processing is useful to remove species from non-clarified wastewaters and when the concentration of the pollutant is extremely low. In this technology, a solid matrix containing the ionic liquid acts as the medium for mass transfer. Ion-exchange technique consists in the exchange of ions in solution with the counterions of the same charge contained in insoluble synthetic polymers or solid matrix.

In: Chemistry Research Summaries Volume 12
Editor: Lucille Monaco Cacioppo
ISBN: 978-1-61668-757-1
© 2014 Nova Science Publishers, Inc.

Chapter 35

APPLICATIONS OF IONIC LIQUIDS IN SAMPLE EXTRACTION

Yunchang Fan[1] and Yan Zhu[2]

[1] College of Physics and Chemistry,
Henan Polytechnic University, Jiaozuo, China
[2] Department of Chemistry, Xixi Campus,
Zhejiang University, Hangzhou, China

RESEARCH SUMMARY

Ionic liquids (ILs), being composed entirely of ions, have become very popular in the last years, because they have many fascinating properties, such as low vapor pressure, low combustibility, excellent thermal stability and wide liquid regions. Extraction is a good approach to reduce the complexity of real samples and concentrate target analytes. This review focuses on the recent progress in the applications of ILs based extraction methods such as liquid phase (micro) extraction and solid phase (micro) extraction in sample extraction field. The advantages and disadvantages of every ILs based sample extraction technique and the future trends about ILs based extraction methods were discussed.

In: Chemistry Research Summaries Volume 12
Editor: Lucille Monaco Cacioppo

ISBN: 978-1-61668-757-1
© 2014 Nova Science Publishers, Inc.

Chapter 36

Ionic Liquid-Based Surfactants

Verónica Pino*, Mónica Germán-Hernández and Armide Martín-Pérez

Department of Analytical Chemistry, Nutrition and Food Science,
University of La Laguna, Spain

Research Summary

Ionic liquids (ILs) are a class of low melting point, ionic compounds which have a variety of properties allowing many of them to be sustainable green solvents. These non-molecular solvents possess high thermal stabilities and negligible vapor pressures making them attractive alternatives to environmentally unfriendly solvents that produce volatile organic compounds (VOCs). Their unique solvation properties, coupled to the fact that they can be structurally tailored for specific applications, have resulted in an increasing study of ILs in many areas of fundamental and applied chemistry.

A new group of ILs able to form aggregates in aqueous solution have been recently described. This behavior makes possible to include these ILs in the category of compounds able to form organized media, like the surfactants. It is very interesting to study these new ILs that exhibit characteristics of cationic surfactants as they constitute a new area of surfactant development, especially considering the limited number of traditional cationic surfactants. Many of these IL-aggregates also possess low critical micelle concentration (CMC) values, which permits the formation of aggregates using smaller amounts of IL. The use of low amounts of ILs also results of environmental interest.

The evaluation of the interaction of dissolved analytes with aqueous pseudophases such as IL-based micelles is a focus of interest. The solubility of hydrophobic compounds can be significantly increased by the presence of IL-based micelles in solution, and this phenomenon has important implications in the development of applications in analytical chemistry as well as in several industrial processes. Obtaining micelle partition coefficients for different classes of analytes (such as drugs or toxic compounds) is of considerable relevance due to the fact that micelles have long been recognized as simple chemical models for biomembranes. Indeed, micelles are structurally more similar to biomembranes than *n*-octanol. The solubilization of analytes into micelles closely resembles that of lipidic bilayers. The influence of several organic solvents on micelles has been studied to understand the effect of solvent perturbation on biological systems. In this sense, it results of interest the obtaining of partition coefficients of different analytes to IL-based micelles.

To sum up, aqueous aggregates of certain ILs can act as adequate substitutes of organic solvents usually employed in conventional extraction processes. Indeed, several works have reported recently the utilization of aqueous IL-based aggregates as extractant solvents in extraction procedures, with improved performance over conventional procedures which utilize large amounts of organic solvents.

In: Chemistry Research Summaries Volume 12
Editor: Lucille Monaco Cacioppo

ISBN: 978-1-61668-757-1
© 2014 Nova Science Publishers, Inc.

Chapter 37

IONIC LIQUIDS IN LIQUID CHROMATOGRAPHY

Hongdeng Qiu[1,2], Abul K. Mallik[1], Makoto Takafuji[1],
Shengxiang Jiang[2] and Hirotaka Ihara[1,*]
[1]Department of Applied Chemistry and Biochemistry,
Kumamoto University, Kumamoto, Japan
[2]Lanzhou Institute of Chemical Physics, Chinese Academy of Science,
Lanzhou, China

RESEARCH SUMMARY

Ionic liquids (ILs) as a new kind of media or materials have been widely studied in broad fields such as material science, catalysis, electrochemistry and analytical chemistry. Interests for ILs in academic and industrial technologies are still increasing due to their unusual chemical and physical properties. In separation science, ionic liquids have been used as extraction media, as mobile phase additives in high-performance liquid chromatography (HPLC), as buffer modifiers in capillary electrophoresis (CE), as stationary phases of gas chromatography (GC) and HPLC, etc. In this chapter, the general physicochemical characters of ILs will be introduced simply and a brief overview of recent developments of ILs in separation science is provided, with a special focus on their use as mobile phase additives and silica-supported IL stationary phases in liquid chromatography.

---

* Fax: +81-96-342-3662; Tel: 81-96-342-3661; E-mail: ihara@kumamoto-u.ac.jp

In: Chemistry Research Summaries Volume 12　　　　ISBN: 978-1-61668-757-1
Editor: Lucille Monaco Cacioppo　　　　© 2014 Nova Science Publishers, Inc.

Chapter 38

IONIC LIQUID IMMOBILIZED NANOPOROUS MATERIALS

Sang-Eon Park and Mst. Nargis Parvin*

National Laboratory of Nano-Green Catalysis and Nano Center for Fine Chemicals
Fusion Technology, Department of Chemistry, Inha University, Incheon, Korea

RESEARCH SUMMARY

Ionic liquids are organic inorganic multi component materials whose chemical (polarity / acidity / co-ordination ability / solubility) and physical (fluidity / conductivity / transferability / liquidus range) properties can be tailored by modifying /changing the type of cations, modifying the alkyl substance in the cations, or modifying / changing the type and the composition of the anions. Ionic liquids have attracted extensive interest in recent years as environmentally benign solvent due to their favorable properties, such as nonflammability, negligible vapor pressure, reusability, high thermal stability and chemical stability. Over the past few years, a variety of catalytic reactions have been successfully conducted using ionic liquids as solvents as well as catalyst. Many interesting results have been obtained, which have demonstrated the advantages of using ILs as the alternatives for organic solvents. Recent development of ionic liquids such as imidazolium based ionic liquids lead the investigations systematically in physical chemistry and in environmental studies as green catalysis. Nowadays both nanoparticles and ionic liquids have become the source of great achievements for the materials chemistry as a heterogeneous organocatalyst. Since the homogeneous reaction systems require a large amount of ionic liquids which is undesirable in the view points of economic and environment. Another problem is the toxicity and viscosity when they are used in bulk. This feature article aims to highlight the main milestones for the better and promising interaction towards nanoparticles and ionic liquids. Two methods, direct co-condensation and post-synthesis-grafting are used for the surface functionalization through microwave or hydrothermal way to prepare heterogeneous organocatalyst. The heterogeneous organocatalyst exhibited a great extent of enhanced catalytic activities for Knoevenagal condensation, Diels-Alder reaction, Henry reaction, Aldol condensation, oxidation of alcohol and alkene. These heterogeneous organocatalysts effectively improved their catalytic applications and performance both in conventional heating and microwave irradiation in various organic syntheses. The combination of supported reagents and microwave irradiation can be used to carry out a wide range of reactions for organic synthesis in short times and with high conversions and selectivity, without solvents. This approach can prove beneficial since the recovery of solvents from conventional reaction systems always results in some losses. This is an emergent awareness of the environmental impact of man-made chemicals.

In: Chemistry Research Summaries Volume 12
Editor: Lucille Monaco Cacioppo

ISBN: 978-1-61668-757-1
© 2014 Nova Science Publishers, Inc.

Chapter 39

ROLES OF IONIC LIQUIDS IN HIGH PERFORMANCE LIQUID CHROMATOGRAPHY

Aurora Martín Calero, Verónica Pino, Juan H. Ayala and Ana M. Afonso*

Department of Analytical Chemistry, Nutrition and Food Science,
University of La Laguna, Spain

RESEARCH SUMMARY

Ionic liquids (ILs) are a class of non-molecular ionic solvents with low melting points resulting from combinations of organic cations and various anions. ILs have many unique properties including wide viscosity ranges, almost negligible vapor pressure, high thermal stability, and a multitude of varying solvation interactions. These outstanding properties justify the high number of applications of these novel solvents in different fundamental and application areas, including analytical sciences.

High-performance liquid-chromatography (HPLC) is a powerful analytical technique in which ILs have also found a variety of applications. The separation of basic compounds in HPLC still remains problematic due to the silanol interactions. The poor performance seen with basic compounds has been partially addressed through the development and introduction of the so-called base-deactivated materials. Nevertheless, addition of alkylamines (such as triethylamine) and other amino quenchers to the mobile phase does not fully remove the deleterious effect of free silanols on the retention of basic analytes, even when employing the purified and least acidic silica supports.

ILs have been proposed as a new alternative to reduce or suppress the silanol effects by using them as organic modifiers in HPLC mobiles phases. The main disadvantage of utilizing pure ILs as organic modifiers is related with their high viscosity. The pressures achieved in the HPLC are normally high when using non-functionalized ILs, even at low flows. In addition to this, ILs are normally expensive, and the consumption of mobiles phases is usually high in HPLC.

For the above mentioned reasons, main uses of ILs in mobile phases of HPLC have been carried out as mobile phase additives, as an alternative to conventional alkyl amines or other amino quenchers. In this field of application, ILs have proven to be much better silanol suppressors than conventional additives.

Finally, ILs have also been proposed as stationary phases in HPLC. ILs have been chemically bonded to the silica support, resulting in a new type of stationary phase. Those packing materials have successfully been used in the separation of inorganic anions, some alkaloids, vitamins and organic acids. The purpose of this kind of stationary phases is also to be able to suppress the silanol effect of conventional stationary phases.

This chapter will focus on the potential applications of ILs as organic modifiers, as mobile phase additives, and as surface-bonded stationary phases in HPLC.

In: Chemistry Research Summaries Volume 12
Editor: Lucille Monaco Cacioppo

ISBN: 978-1-61668-757-1
© 2014 Nova Science Publishers, Inc.

Chapter 40

THE UNIQUE PHYSICAL AND CHEMICAL PROPERTIES OF IONIC LIQUIDS THROUGH INTERIONIC INTERACTIONS: THEORETICAL INVESTIGATION WITH MOLECULAR DYNAMICS SIMULATIONS

*Tateki Ishida**

Department of Theoretical and Computational Molecular Science
Institute for Molecular Science, Japan

RESEARCH SUMMARY

Ionic liquids (ILs) have been found to possess a wide potential variety of interesting physical and chemical properties. We consider here the unique properties of ILs, which owe to the specific interionic interaction between ionic species. In particular, we discuss the importance of both the cross-correlation between cation and anion species and the effect of polarization in ILs. Based on recent theoretical studies on ILs employing molecular dynamics simulations, how the collective dynamics through interionic interactions cause the unique physical and chemical properties of ILs and how electronic polarizability effects modify interionic dynamics are presented. The former includes the investigation of the contribution of ionic motions due to Coulombic interactions to velocity cross-correlation functions, analyzing the longitudinal and nonlongitudinal motions in ILs, and the study of many-body polarization effects on the cage effect in ILs. The latter discusses the relation between polarizability correlation functions and interionic interactions, considering the Kerr spectra of ILs. Also, some of the theoretical backgrounds for studying the cross-correlation between ionic species are summarized, and the theoretical and computational procedures for treating polarization effect on ILs with molecular dynamics simulations are given.

* E-mail: ishida@ims.ac.jp

In: Chemistry Research Summaries Volume 12
Editor: Lucille Monaco Cacioppo

ISBN: 978-1-61668-757-1
© 2014 Nova Science Publishers, Inc.

Chapter 41

Ionic Liquid-Solid Interface Probed by Scanning Tunneling Microscopy

Ge-Bo Pan[*], Yong-Qiang Liu and Yan Xiao

Suzhou Institute of Nano-tech and Nano-bionics,
Chinese Academy of Sciences, Suzhou, China

Research Summary

In this chapter, we have reviewed the current state of the knowledge of the ionic liquid-solid interface, which is vital for applications and whose studies are still in its infancy. Emphasis has been placed on atomic or molecular-resolution characterization by scanning tunneling microscopy (STM). Firstly, technological point of STM for ionic liquids (ILs) has been briefly discussed. Secondly, updated researches on the adsorption behavior of anions and cations of ILs are exploited. Thirdly, potentials of ILs in metal deposition are reviewed. Fourthly, potentials of ILs in deposition of elemental and compound semiconductors are discussed. Finally, applications of ILs in deposition of organic molecules are briefly discussed. We conclude this chapter with personal perspectives on the directions to which future research on this field might be directed.

---

[*] Corresponding authors. Fax: +86-512-62872663. E-mail address: gbpan2008@sinano.ac.cn

In: Chemistry Research Summaries Volume 12 ISBN: 978-1-61668-757-1
Editor: Lucille Monaco Cacioppo © 2014 Nova Science Publishers, Inc.

Chapter 42

ENZYMATIC CATALYSIS IN BUFFERED IONIC LIQUIDS

Guangnan Ou

School of Bioengineering, Jimei University,
Xiamen, P.R. China

RESEARCH SUMMARY

Many chemical reactions are sensitive to pH values, that is, the yield of products and even the nature of the products may be altered appreciably if the pH changes significantly during the process of reaction. This is especially true in biochemical reactions where the pH is important to the proper metabolism and functioning of animals and plants. We can efficiently control the pH of an aqueous media at a predetermined level by the addition of water-soluble buffer substances. In non-aqueous media, common buffers were found to have only limited solubility, therefore, reactions in non-aqueous media have been investigated without controlling the pH of the system. To overcome this restriction, we have designed and synthesized a new class of ionic liquid (IL) with buffering behaviour that are referred to as IL buffers, which are miscible with polar solvents such as methanol, DMF, and dichloromethane and also with ILs like [BMIM][PF_6] and [BMIM][BF_4]. For the development of buffered enzymatic ionic liquid systems, ionic-liquid buffer having phosphate anion was synthesized. The effects of IL and buffer on activity and stability of *Candida antarctica* lipase B (CALB) were investigated using the transesterification of ethyl butyrate with n-butanol as a model reaction. Fluorometric measurements were applied to analyze changes in enzyme conformation to understand the activation and denaturation phenomena of the dissolved enzyme in IL media. The results showed that both the conformation and transesterification activity of CALB dissolved in the hydroxyl-functionalized ionic liquids were buffer dependent. Intrinsic fluorescence studies indicated that the CALB possessed a more compact conformation in the medium consisted of ionic liquid buffer having phosphate anion and hydroxyl-functionalized ionic liquids like 1-(1-hydroxyethyl)-3-methyl-imidazolium tetrafluoroborate and 1-(1-hydroxyethyl)-3-methyl-imidazolium nitrate. High activity and outstanding stability could be obtained with the buffered enzymatic ionic liquid systems for the transesterification. We proposed a plausible theoretical hypothesis based on ionizing and dissociating properties to give a deeper understanding of enzyme catalysis in buffered ionic liquids.

In: Chemistry Research Summaries Volume 12
Editor: Lucille Monaco Cacioppo

ISBN: 978-1-61668-757-1
© 2014 Nova Science Publishers, Inc.

Chapter 43

PREPARATION OF FUNCTIONAL ION GELS OF POLYSACCHARIDES WITH IONIC LIQUIDS

*Jun-ichi Kadokawa**

Graduate School of Science and Engineering,
Kagoshima University, Kagoshima, Japan

RESEARCH SUMMARY

Ionic liquids, which are low-melting point salts and form liquids at room temperature or the temperatures below the boiling point of water, have recently received significant attention as the solvents in a wide range of the research fields, such as separation and reaction media. Ionic liquids have been used as good solvents for natural polysaccharides such as cellulose and chitin. This chapter describes the preparation of functional ion gels of the polysaccharides with ionic liquids, which include the ionic liquids as the disperse media in the polysaccharide network matrixes. When the cellulose solution in an ionic liquid, 1-butyl-3-methylimidazolium chloride (BMIMCl) was left standing at room temperature for 7 days, it gradually became the gel form. The resulting ion gel was characterized by the elemental analysis, TGA, and XRD measurements, which suggested that the gel was obtained by formation of the cellulose aggregates as cross-linking points in the solution owing to gradually absorbing water into the solution. This gelling technique was extended to provide ion gels of cellulose/starch and cellulose/chitin composite systems. Furthermore, the preparation of ion gels of hydrocolloid polysaccharides, such as carrageenan, xanthan gum, and guar gum, with BMIMCl was also achieved. The resulting ion gels exhibited specific unique and high performance properties.

---

* Tel: +81-99-285-7743, Fax: +81-99-285-3253, E-mail: kadokawa@eng.kagoshima-u.ac.jp

In: Chemistry Research Summaries Volume 12
Editor: Lucille Monaco Cacioppo

ISBN: 978-1-61668-757-1
© 2014 Nova Science Publishers, Inc.

Chapter 44

THE APPLICATION OF IONIC LIQUIDS-CELLULOSE HYDROLYSIS TO CHEMICALS

*Furong Tao[1,2], Huanling Song[1] and Lingjun Chou[1]**

[1]State Key Laboratory for Oxo Synthesis and Selective Oxidation, Lanzhou Institute of Chemical Physics, Chinese Academy of Sciences, Lanzhou, P. R. China
[2]Graduate School of Chinese Academy of Sciences, Beijing, P. R. China

RESEARCH SUMMARY

The efficient utilization of biomass has recently received considerable attention as a potential alternative to petroleum for the production of transportation fuels and chemicals. Cellulose, which is the most abundant natural polymeric carbon source in the word, occupies 30-40% of biomass. Until now, studies have mainly focus on the efficient depolymerization of cellulose into small molecular platform chemicals, because cellulose itself is a highly crystalline polymer of D-anhydroglucopyranose units jointed together in long chains by β-1,4-glycosidic bonds. The tight hydrogen bonding network and van der Waals interactions greatly stabilize cellulose, making it notoriously resistant to hydrolysis.

Ionic liquids (ILs), which have some specific properties (such as non-volatility, non-flammability, low toxicity, biodegradability, high thermal and chemical stability, etc.), are attracting increasing attention as a new "green" solvent. It is these characteristic which lead to an explosion in their use in a wide range of catalytic and stoichiometric reactions as well as in many other applications. Based on the fact that cellulose is hardly soluble in conventional solvents because of its intermolecular hydrogen bonds, and many studies have shown that cellulose can be dissolved in some hydrophilic ILs, catalytic hydrolysis of cellulose to chemicals in ionic liquids has received significant attention in recent years.

Our promising biomass-derived platform chemicals are 5-hydroxymethylfurfural (HMF) and furfural, which are suitable for alternative polymers or for liquid biofuels. Currently, HMF can be produced from glucose and fructose, the ability to generate HMF and furfural directly from cellulose would remove a major barrier. Here we report a single-step catalytic

---

* Corresponding author: Fax: +86 931 4968129; Tel: +86 931 4968066; E-mail address: ljchou@licp.cas.cn

process where cellulose was rapidly hydrolyzed in ionic liquids and the resulting glucose was converted to HMF and furfural under mild conditions. Biphasic systems were used in our study, in which water-immiscible organic solvent methylisobutylketone (MIBK) was added to extract continuously the main products from the aqueous phase. The schematic illustration of productions from cellulose was shown in scheme 1.

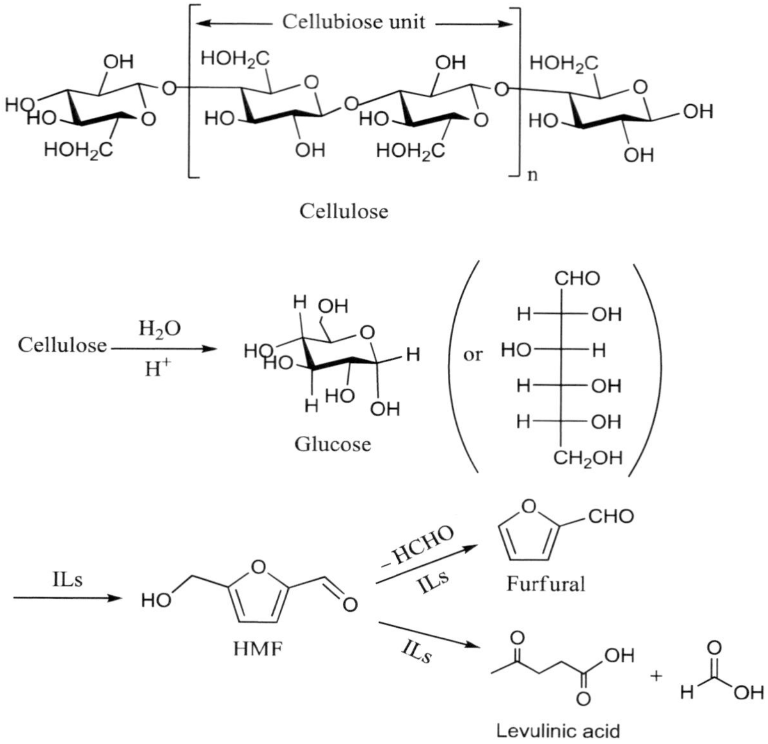

Scheme 1. The schematic illustration of productions from cellulose.

In: Chemistry Research Summaries Volume 12
Editor: Lucille Monaco Cacioppo

ISBN: 978-1-61668-757-1
© 2014 Nova Science Publishers, Inc.

Chapter 45

Separation of Aromatic and Organic Nitrogen Compounds with Supported Ionic Liquid Membranes

Michiaki Matsumoto

Department of Chemical Engineering and Materials Science,
Doshisha University, Kyotanabe, Kyoto, Japan

Research Summary

Aromatic hydrocarbons and organic nitrogen compounds were separated with supported liquid membranes using ionic liquids, based on 1-alkyl-3-methylimidazorium and quaternary ammonium salts. The aromatic hydrocarbons and organic nitrogen compounds selectively permeated the membranes. Liquid membranes that used more hydrophilic ionic liquids yielded higher selectivity. The ionic liquids were retained in membrane pores after ten times repeated experiments. Supported liquid membranes based on ionic liquids were applied to separation of aromatic hydrocarbons, organic nitrogen and sulfur compounds from model fuels. These compounds were successfully permeated through the membranes. Supported ionic liquid membranes were found to be promising technique for separating polar organic compounds.

In: Chemistry Research Summaries Volume 12
Editor: Lucille Monaco Cacioppo

ISBN: 978-1-61668-757-1
© 2014 Nova Science Publishers, Inc.

Chapter 46

IONIC LIQUIDS IN EXTRACTION TECHNIQUES

N. Fontanals, E. Pocurull, R. M. Marcé[*] and F. Borrull
Universitat Rovira i Virgili, Department of Analytical Chemistry
and Organic Chemistry, Tarragona, Spain

RESEARCH SUMMARY

Ionic liquids (ILs) have high polarity, very low miscibility with water, negligible vapor pressure, high thermal stability and relatively high viscosity. All of these features make them good polar solvents for a wide range of compounds. Consequently, ILs have attracted interest as green solvents for chemical processes, including organic synthesis, and chemical analyses, in which they have been used in both separation and extraction techniques.

This chapter reviews the application of ILs in a variety of extraction techniques. It describes how ILs can be used as solvents or modifiers in liquid-liquid extraction, liquid-phase microextraction, single-drop microextraction, hollow-fiber liquid-phase microextraction or solid-phase microextraction, among other techniques, or how they can be part of stationary phases, in such sorptive techniques as solid-phase microextraction and solid-phase extraction. The use of ILs as part of extraction techniques for solid samples such as ultrasonically assisted extraction and microwave-assisted extraction will also be reviewed. The type and role of ILs used in these extraction techniques and their advantages and drawbacks will be discussed. Representative examples of the applications of each extraction technique will also be given.

[*] Universitat Rovira i Virgili , Department of Analytical Chemistry and Organic Chemistry, Sescelades Campus, Marcel·lí Domingo s/n, 43007-Tarragona (Spain), Tel: 34 977 558170, Fax: 34 977 558446, *E-mail: rosamaria.marce@urv.cat

In: Chemistry Research Summaries Volume 12
Editor: Lucille Monaco Cacioppo

ISBN: 978-1-61668-757-1
© 2014 Nova Science Publishers, Inc.

Chapter 47

SURFACE-ACTIVE IONIC LIQUIDS: SYNTHESES, SOLUTION PROPERTIES, AND APPLICATIONS

Paula D. Galgano and Omar A. El Seoud[*]

Institute of Chemistry, University of São Paulo, São Paulo, S.P., Brazil

RESEARCH SUMMARY

The highly favorable properties of ionic liquids, ILs, e.g., negligible vapor pressure; high polarity; high chemical and thermal stability, as well as molecular structural versatility are expected to be carried over to their surface-active counterparts, SAILs, (ILs with long-chain "tails"); this has been verified experimentally for several 1,3-dialkylimidazolium electrolytes (e.g., chlorides, bromides, and tetrafluoroborates). The impetus for studying SAILs is the enormous potential for their applications, e.g., in the nano-technological and biomedical fields. The progress in these applications rests on a clear understanding of the relationship between surfactant molecular structure and properties. This review article is focused on imidazole-based SAILs, including: syntheses, determination of the properties of their solutions; comparison between their micellar properties and those of "conventional" cationic surfactants, and their main applications. The most frequently employed schemes for the synthesis and purification of SAILs are given; the following micellar properties are listed, *where available*: the critical micelles concentrations, counter-ion dissociation constants; surfactant aggregation numbers; thermodynamic parameters of aggregation. Where possible, we compare the above-mentioned properties with those of "conventional" surfactants in order to show the relevance to aggregation of the imidazolium ring. The above-mentioned applications are briefly discussed.

[*] Institute of Chemistry, University of São Paulo, P. O. Box 26077, 05513-970, São Paulo, S.P., Brazil, Fax: 55-11-3091-3874; E-mail: elseoud@iq.usp.br

In: Chemistry Research Summaries Volume 12
Editor: Lucille Monaco Cacioppo

ISBN: 978-1-61668-757-1
© 2014 Nova Science Publishers, Inc.

Chapter 48

THE APPLICATION OF IONIC
LIQUIDS IN POLYCONDENSATION

Liu Zhengping, Wang Jing, Peng Qiaohong and Yin Zuo

College of Chemistry, BNU Key Lab of Environmentally Friendly and Functional
Polymer Materials, Beijing Normal University, Beijing, China

RESEARCH SUMMARY

Polycondensation is one of the main polymerizations for preparing polymers, especially the engineering plastics including Poly(ethylene terephthalate)(PET), Polyamide(PA), Polyimide(PI), Polycarbonate(PC) which are widely used in our daily life. The polymerization procedure usually needs high temperature, high billing point organic solvent, high vacuum and small molecular motivation to promote equilibrium move. So it seems reasonable to introduce ionic liquids into polycondensation due to their low volatility, high thermal stability, possibility of recycling, environmentally friendly, and so on. The application of ionic liquids as solvents, catalysts, and monomers in polycondensation is the subject of this chapter.

In: Chemistry Research Summaries Volume 12
Editor: Lucille Monaco Cacioppo

ISBN: 978-1-61668-757-1
© 2014 Nova Science Publishers, Inc.

Chapter 49

PHASE EQUILIBRIA IN THE FULLERENE-CONTAINING SYSTEMS

Konstantin N. Semenov[1], *Nikolay A. Charykov*
[1] St. Petersburg State University, St. Petersburg, Russia

RESEARCH SUMMARY

Experimental and literature data concerning different types of phase equilibria (liquid-solid, liquid-liquid and sorption equilibria) in the fullerene-containing systems are presented and discussed, as well as application of investigated systems in medicine, pharmacology, food, cosmetic industry and for pre-chromatographic separation of the light fullerenes industrial mixtures.

In: Chemistry Research Summaries Volume 12
Editor: Lucille Monaco Cacioppo

ISBN: 978-1-61668-757-1
© 2014 Nova Science Publishers, Inc.

Chapter 50

IONIC COMPOUNDS OF FULLERENES OBTAINED BY SYNTHESIS IN SOLUTION

D. V. Konarev, R. N. Lyubovskaya
Institute of Problems of Chemical Physics RAS
Chernogolovka, Russia

RESEARCH SUMMARY

In this review we discuss the current state in the field of the design and study of ionic fullerene compounds with organic and organometallic donors as well as organic and metal-containing cations, which are obtained by direct synthesis from solution as single crystals or polycrystals. We summarize the data on transformations of fullerene anions associated with their dimerization, polymerization or coordination and discuss the effect of these processes on the properties of ionic compounds. Ionic fullerene complexes with magnetic transitions, metallic conductivity and coexistence of high conductivity and magnetic interactions are also discussed.

In: Chemistry Research Summaries Volume 12
Editor: Lucille Monaco Cacioppo

ISBN: 978-1-61668-757-1
© 2014 Nova Science Publishers, Inc.

Chapter 51

SYMMETRICAL FEATURES OF THE FULLERENE STRUCTURES IN THE LIGHT OF FUNDAMENTAL DOMAINS THEORY OF POINT SYMMETRY GROUPS

V. M. Talanov and N. V. Fedorova

South Russian State Technical University,
(Novocherkassk Polytechnic Institute),
Novocherkassk, Russia

RESEARCH SUMMARY

In the review the bases of the original geometrical theory of fundamental domains of three-dimensional point groups of symmetry and results of application of this theory to research of symmetrical and structural features of fullerenes are stated.

A fundamental domain of symmetry group is called the part of space, images of which cover all space without admissions and self-crossings under the action of group symmetry operations.

Structural elements of fundamental regions are characterized by certain own symmetry and orbits symmetry, special geometrical properties and interrelation with each other. They also have certain own structure: tops, edges, sides and three-dimensional components. Classification of structural elements of fundamental regions of point groups is made. Isosymmetrical, enantiomorphical, antiisostructural, extraordinary, exclusive and irrational structural elements are stated.

Structural elements of fundamental domains of point groups of symmetry are geometrical images of symmetrical states in which there can be molecules as a result of lowering of their symmetry. Lowering of molecules symmetry can be connected with the change of external conditions, internal structural regroupings, doping, replacements of atoms and other reasons. Therefore geometrical interrelation between structural elements of fundamental domains reflects possible ways of structural transformations of molecules and allows us to specify conditions of a continuity of structural transformations. Graphs of adjacency of structural elements of fundamental domains of point groups have been constructed with this purpose.

The geometrical theory offered allows us to state symmetrical and structural features of fullerene $C_{60,}$ C_{20}, C_{24}, C_{28}, C_{40}, C_{48} and C_{56}.

In: Chemistry Research Summaries Volume 12 ISBN: 978-1-61668-757-1
Editor: Lucille Monaco Cacioppo © 2014 Nova Science Publishers, Inc.

Chapter 52

BIOMEDICAL APPLICATION OF FULLERENES

Vukosava Milic Torres[1], Branislava Srdjenovic[2]

[1]National Institute of Health Dr. Ricardo Jorge,
Department of Genetics, Laboratory of Proteomics, Lisbon, Portugal
[2]Medical Faculty, Department of Pharmacy,
University of Novi Sad, Novi Sad, Republic of Serbia

RESEARCH SUMMARY

Fullerene, the third carbon allotrope, is a classical engineered material with the potential application in biomedicine. Since their discovery in 1985, fullerenes have been extensively investigated. The biological activities of fullerenes are considerably influenced by their chemical modifications and light treatment. The most relevant feature of fullerene C_{60} is the ability to act as a free radical scavenges. Properties attributed to the delocalized π double bond system of fullerene cage allow C_{60} to quench various free radicals more efficiently than conventional antioxidants. However, extremely high hydrophobicity of fullerene hampers its direct biomedical evaluation and application. To overcome this problem, several approaches for the transfer fullerenes into physiological friendly media have been developed: chemical modification of the fullerene carbon cage, incorporation of fullerenes into water soluble micellar supramolecular structures, solvent exchange and long term stirring of pure C_{60} in water. These steps created army of different classes of functionalized fullerenes which exhibit vast range of biological activities, especially in the field of photodynamic therapy, neuroprotection, apoptosis, drug and gene delivery. It was found that certain classes of functionalized fullerenes can be used for diagnostic purposes. So far, the most promising applications include the use of gadolinium endohedral complexes in magnetic resonance imaging and therpautic (as a primary or adjuvant) exploration of tris-adducts and polyhidroxlated C_{60} fullerenes. In this chapter we are summarizing and discussing main biological and medicinal aspects of fullerenes and its functionalized derivates with special regards to the recent achievements.

In: Chemistry Research Summaries Volume 12   ISBN: 978-1-61668-757-1
Editor: Lucille Monaco Cacioppo   © 2014 Nova Science Publishers, Inc.

Chapter 53

METAL COMPLEX CATALYSIS IN THE CHEMISTRY OF FULLERENES

Usein M. Dzhemilev and Airat R. Tuktarov

Institute of Petrochemistry and Catalysis of Russian Academy of Sciences,
Ufa, Bashkortostan, Russian Federation

RESEARCH SUMMARY

This chapter surveys the published data on the use of metal complex catalysts in the synthesis of functionally substituted fullerenes.

The review considers various reactions of fullerenes, in particular, radical reactions, the reactions with electrophilic and nucleophilic reagents and small molecules using metal complex catalysts.

In some cases, thermal and catalytic methods for fullerene functionalization are presented to demonstrate the advantages of catalytic reactions. The mechanisms of formation of the target cluster compounds and the possible applications of the functionally substituted fullerenes are discussed.

In: Chemistry Research Summaries Volume 12
Editor: Lucille Monaco Cacioppo

ISBN: 978-1-61668-757-1
© 2014 Nova Science Publishers, Inc.

Chapter 54

DFT STUDY OF FULLERENOL AND FULLERENOL-LIKE INORGANIC MOLECULES AND IONS SUCCESSIVELY SUBSTITUTED BY ALKALI METAL ATOMS

Oleg P. Charkin[1,*], *Nina M. Klimenko*[2,#], *Yi-Sheng Wang*[3,†]

[1] Institute of Problems of Chemical Physics,
Russian Academy of Sciences,
Chernogolovka, Moscow oblast, Russia
[2] Lomonosov State Academy of Fine Chemical Technology,
Moscow, Russia
[3] Genomics Research Center, Academia Sinica,
Nankang, Taipei, Taiwan

RESEARCH SUMMARY

The equilibrium geometric parameters and the energetic characteristics of fullerenol molecules and ions $C_{60}(OH)_{24-n}(OL)_n$ and $C_{60}(OH)_{24-n}(OL)_nL^+$ substituted successively by alkali metal atoms L with the number of substitutions $n = 1 - 24$, have been calculated by the density functional B3LYP/6-31G* method. Computations have shown that the first four single substitutions of Li for H in the OH groups attached to the same C_6 benzenoid ring require very low energy inputs (less than 1 kcal/mol), and can spontaneously occur under common conditions. The further fifth and sixth single substitutions in the same C_6 ring are endothermic, but the required energy inputs are also modest ($2 - 5$ kcal/mol). The first and second "cooperative" substitutions of Li for H simultaneously in all four hydroxylated C_6 rings require energy inputs of ~ 2.5 and ~ 9 kcal/mol, respectively; in the third and fourth fourfold substitutions, the energies increase up to ~15.5 kcal/mol. The mean partial energy

[*] E-mail address: charkin@icp.ac.ru
[#] E-mail address: nmklimenko@mitht.ru
[†] E-mail address: wer@gate.sinica.edu.tw

per single substitution of Li for H averaged over this series ($n = 1 - 6$) does not exceed $\sim 2.0 -$ 2.5 kcal/mol. It is predicted that isolated $C_{60}(OH)_{24 - n}(OLi)_n$ molecules and corresponding ions with intermediate number of substitution ($n = 1 - 16$) can be formed under the conditions of relatively low energy inputs (for example, under the conditions of the MALDI experiment). For the sodium- and potassium-substituted analogues, the qualitative pattern persists, but the H/Na and H/K substitutions are somewhat more endothermic. The computational results are compared with MALDI mass spectrum of the $[C_{60}(OH)_x(ONa)_y +$ $CH_3COONa]$ system in which series of the substituted positive ions $C_{60}(OH)_x(ONa)_y^+$ ($x + y =$ 24) were detected with y rising up to 13. Similar semiquantitative picture was found in the calculations of related $C_{60}(OH)_{20 - n}(OLi)_n$ and $C_{60}(OH)_{18 - n}(OLi)_n$ fullerenols.

For comparison, the B3LYP/6-31G* calculations have been performed for a few fullerenol-like substituted inorganic cages like the icosahedral $B_{12}(OH)_{12 - n}(OLi)_n^{2-}$ and dodecahedral $Si_{20}O_{30}(OH)_{20 - n}(OLi)_n$ $Ti_{20}O_{30}(OH)_{20 - n}(OLi)_n$ clusters, where H/Li substitutions were predicted to be moderately exothermic and to proceed more easy and completely, than those for the fullerenols.

In: Chemistry Research Summaries Volume 12
Editor: Lucille Monaco Cacioppo

ISBN: 978-1-61668-757-1
© 2014 Nova Science Publishers, Inc.

Chapter 55

HOW TO IMPROVE THE PROPERTIES OF POLYMER MEMBRANES: MODIFICATION OF MEMBRANE MATERIALS BY CARBON NANOPARTICLES

A. V. Penkova[1,*] *and G. A. Polotskaya* [1,2]

[1] Saint-Petersburg State University,
Department of Chemical Thermodynamics & Kinetics,
Universitetsky pr. 26, Petrodvoretz, Saint-Petersburg, Russia
[2] Institute of Macromolecular Compounds,
Russian Academy of Sciences, Saint-Petersburg, Russia

RESEARCH SUMMARY

Polymer modification by carbon nanoparticles is a way for the development of new membrane materials. Composites of poly(phenylene isophtalamide) (PA) with fullerene C_{60} and carbon nanotubes (CNT) were developed and used for preparation of asymmetric and homogeneous membranes. Character of interaction between PA and carbon particles in composites was studied by spectroscopic methods. The effect of carbon particles inclusion in PA matrix on some physical properties was estimated. Scanning electron microscopy was employed in visualizing internal morphology of the both asymmetric and homogeneous membranes. Transport properties of homogeneous membranes based on pure PA and its composites containing 2, 5, and 10 wt% C_{60} or CNT were studied in pervaporation of methanol-containing mixtures (methanol/cyclohexane and methanol/ methyl tert-butyl ether). The effect of carbon additives (fullerene, cabon nanotubes, or graphite soot) on the performance of PA asymmetric membranes was examined in ultrafiltration. Membranes were tested in separation of 0.4 wt% mixture of proteins with various molecular weights in aqueous solution. It was established that modification of membrane materials by carbon particles such as fullerene C_{60} and nanotubes leads to improvement of transport properties in pervaporation and ultrafiltration.

---

* E-mail address: anast.chem@gmail.com

In: Chemistry Research Summaries Volume 12
Editor: Lucille Monaco Cacioppo

ISBN: 978-1-61668-757-1
© 2014 Nova Science Publishers, Inc.

Chapter 56

FUNCTIONALIZED NANOFULLERENES FOR HYDROGEN STORAGE: A THEORETICAL PERSPECTIVE

N. S. Venkataramanan[1,2,*], *A. Suvitha*[2], *H. Mizuseki*[2], *and Y. Kawazoe*[2]

[1] College of Science, California State University,
Hayward, California, US
[2] Institute for Materials Research (IMR),
Tohoku University, Katahira, Aoba-ku, Sendai, Japan

RESEARCH SUMMARY

The increase in threats from global warming due to the consumption of fossil fuels requires our planet to adopt new strategies to harness the inexhaustible sources of energy. Hydrogen is an energy carrier which holds tremendous promise as a new renewable and clean energy option. Hydrogen is a convenient, safe, versatile fuel source that can be easily converted to a desired form of energy without releasing harmful emissions. However, no materials was found satisfy the desired goals and hence there is hunt for new materials that can store hydrogen reversibly at ambient conditions. In this chapter, we discuss and compare various nanofullerene materials proposed theoretically as storage medium for hydrogen. Doping of transition elements leads to clustering which reduces the gravimetric density of hydrogen, while doping of alkali and alkali-earth metals on the nanocage materials, such as carborides, boronitride, and boron cages, were stabilized by the charger transfer from the dopant to the nanocage. Further, the alkali or alkali-earth elements exist with a charge, which are found to be responsible for the higher uptake of hydrogen, through a dipole- dipole and change-induced dipole interaction. The binding energies of hydrogen on these systems were found to be in the range of 0.1 eV to 0.2 eV, which are ideal for the practical applications in a reversible system.

---

[*] E-mail address: nsvenkataramanan@gmail.com, ramanan@imr.edu

In: Chemistry Research Summaries Volume 12   ISBN: 978-1-61668-757-1
Editor: Lucille Monaco Cacioppo   © 2014 Nova Science Publishers, Inc.

Chapter 57

SELF-ASSEMBLY PROPERTIES OF FULLERENES

Martin J. Hollamby, Takashi Nakanishi[1]

National Institute for Materials Science (NIMS),
Tsukuba, Japan

RESEARCH SUMMARY

It has long been known that the formation of ordered, long-range assemblies is critical to realize any of the myriad, but mostly quiescent real-world applications of fullerene-containing systems. In a bid to achieve this aim, a wide variety of different approaches have been used, particularly concerned with the formation of well-defined arrays of pristine C_{60} e.g., by liquid-liquid interfacial precipitation, template-assisted dip drying, drop drying, rapid re-precipitation or supramolecular co-assembly. Another arguably simpler method is the chemical functionalization of C_{60} with hydrophilic or hydrophobic moieties, which increase its solubility in common solvents, permitting more facile processing. These derivatized fullerenes can self-organize to form hierarchical structures, including polymorphous aggregates and liquid crystalline assemblies, which exhibit interesting structural and optoelectronic properties. In this review, we summarize the state of the art in this exciting field, with particular emphasis on the development of a macromolecular toolbox to incorporate the benefits of C_{60} into functional materials.

---

[1] e-mail address: Nakanishi.Takashi@nims.go.jp

In: Chemistry Research Summaries Volume 12
Editor: Lucille Monaco Cacioppo
ISBN: 978-1-61668-757-1
© 2014 Nova Science Publishers, Inc.

Chapter 58

[60]FULLERENE AND DERIVATIVES IN BIOLOGY AND MEDICINE

Henri Szwarc and Fathi Moussa[1]
LETIAM EA 4041, IUT d'Orsay, Université Paris, France

RESEARCH SUMMARY

Since the early nineties, hundreds of papers have been devoted to the study of possible uses of [60]fullerene (C_{60}) and its derivatives in the biomedical field. Many applications have been proposed including enzyme inhibition, DNA cleavage, photodynamic therapy, mainly cancer therapy, antiviral activity, free radicals scavenging, etc. In 2004 some publications raised considerable doubt about fullerenes safety, which slowed down the research efforts in this area and partly diverted them towards some fullerene derivatives supposedly less toxic than pristine C_{60}. However, recent studies showed that the alleged dangers of C_{60} were in fact due to the solvent used to prepare colloidal aggregates of this fullerene. Thus, studies on biomedical applications of C_{60} resumed, notably because of its efficiency in the field of oxidative stress. To understand possible biomedical applications of fullerenes, we will first recall some general physical properties of these compounds relevant to this purpose. Specific biological applications of fullerenes are then discussed. A section on toxicity and in vivo fate of C_{60} and derivatives is also included.

---

[1] E-mail address: fathi.moussa@u-psud.fr

In: Chemistry Research Summaries Volume 12
Editor: Lucille Monaco Cacioppo

ISBN: 978-1-61668-757-1
© 2014 Nova Science Publishers, Inc.

Chapter 59

SPECTROSCOPY AND MODELING OF THERMAL STABILITY AND DEFECT STATES IN POLYMER-FULLERENE C_{60} COMPOSITES

A. O. Pozdnyakov[1,2][1], *A. A. Konchits*[3], *A. L. Pushkarchuk*[4]

[1] Institute of Problems of Mechanical Engineering, St. Petersburg, Russia
[2] Ioffe Physico-Technical Institute, St-Petersburg, Russia
[3] V. E. Lashkarev Institute of Semiconductor Physics, Kyiv, Ukraine
[4] Institute of Physical and Organic Chemistry, Minsk, Belarus

RESEARCH SUMMARY

Polymer-fullerene composites prepared by mixing the components are attractive due to simplicity of their preparation. For many applications it is of high importance to control the thermal stability changes of the polymer matrix in the presence of the guest fullerene molecules. Our chapter describes the attempts to understand this problem by using peculiar combination of experimental (mass-spectrometry, electron paramagnetic resonance) and theoretical (quantum chemistry) approaches to study polystyrene-C_{60} and polymethylmethacrylate-C_{60} blends. The results provide molecular level interpretation of the low temperature depolymerization of polymethylmethacrylate macromolecules in the presence of fullerene C_{60} which is not experimentally observed for polystyrene-C_{60} blend. Effect of oxygen in the above processes is outlined.

[1] E-mail address: ao.pozd@mail.ioffe.ru

In: Chemistry Research Summaries Volume 12
Editor: Lucille Monaco Cacioppo

ISBN: 978-1-61668-757-1
© 2014 Nova Science Publishers, Inc.

Chapter 60

EFFECT OF C$_{60}$ DOPING ON THE STRUCTURE AND PROPERTIES OF POLYSTYRENE

Olga V. Alekseeva[1], Nadezhda A. Bagrovskaya[1], Sergey M. Kuzmin[1], Andrew V. Noskov[1], Igor V. Melikhov[2] and Vsevolod. N. Rudin[2]

[1] Institute of Solution Chemistry, Russian Academy of Sciences,
Ivanovo, Russia
[2] Faculty of Chemistry, Moscow State University, Moscow, Russia

RESEARCH SUMMARY

The present chapter includes the detailed study on the structural properties and biological activity of both polystyrene films and polystyrene films containing fullerene. The basic attention is given to kinetics of hierarchical nanostructures formation in surface layer of polystyrene-fullerene composite.

The structural characteristics of polystyrene films modified by the incorporation of fullerenes were researched by the infrared spectroscopy, ultraviolet spectroscopy, and X-ray diffraction technique. According to IR-spectroscopy data it was suggested that intermolecular interaction between polymer's phenyl ring and fullerene molecule occurs in the composite material. Semi quantitative analysis of IR spectra of the studied films with application of a method of a base line and internal standard was carried out. Analysis of UV spectra confirms the assumption that there is the interaction of polystyrene electron-donor molecule with π-electronic system of fullerene.

By the X-ray diffraction technique it is shown that structures with 2.3, 2.5 and 3.9 Å interplanar distances are present in the fullerene doped polystyrene films. The analysis of a small angle area of difractograms evidences fractal structure of studied polystyrene composites.

We have studied a primary aggregates formation stage of polymer molecules in solutions of polystyrene in *o*-xylene containing small amounts of fullerenes. Aggregates formed in a solution layer applied to an inert substrate upon evaporation of the solvent at ambient temperature and conversion of the solution into a polymer film. The film surface was examined under a scanning electron microscope. It is visualized that the surface is composed of spheroids with irregular relief, the size of irregularities being comparable with the polystyrene molecule size (10 nm). From analysis of the size distribution functions we are concluded that formation of primary aggregates can be described as successive addition of polystyrene molecules to the previously formed aggregates, which differ only in size. Continuum approximation turns out to be adequate in a wide range of sizes up to molecular ones. It is follows from the fact that experimental data is consistent with solution of Fokker-Planck-type kinetic equation which is a condition of particles number conservation.

Antimicrobial activity of the polystyrene-fullerene composites was tested against gram-positives (Staphylococcus aureus) and gram-negative (Escherichia coli, Pseudomonas aeruginosa) microorganisms and fungi association. The test results showed absolute death of the microorganisms under the modified film. It should be noted that dynamics of the bacteria inactivation persists during a month.

In: Chemistry Research Summaries Volume 12
Editor: Lucille Monaco Cacioppo

ISBN: 978-1-61668-757-1
© 2014 Nova Science Publishers, Inc.

Chapter 61

1D FULLERENE C$_{60}$ MICRO/NANO FIBERS SYNTHESIZED BY LIQUID-LIQUID INTERFACIAL PRECIPITATION METHOD

Guangzhe Piao[1] and Yongtao Qu

Key Laboratory of Rubber-Plastics, Ministry of Education,
School of Polymer Science and Engineering
Qingdao University of Science and Technology,
Qingdao, China

RESEARCH SUMMARY

C$_{60}$ is a well-known fullerene prototype; zero-dimensional structure has been generally accepted for C$_{60}$ fullerene. Through simple and easy-to-control method, 1D fullerene C$_{60}$ micro/nano fibers (FNFs) were successfully prepared by liquid-liquid interfacial precipitation using toluene, *m*-xylene, pyridine and/or N-methyl-2-pyrrolidone (NMP) as solvents and isopropyl alcohol as precipitation agent. There is a systematic correlation between the type of the solvents and the final structures of the C$_{60}$ FNFs prepared using LLIP. When the solvents were toluene and *m*-xylene, solid C$_{60}$ fullerene nanowhiskers (FNWs) were easily synthesized. On the other hand, the fullerene C$_{60}$ micro/nano tubes (FNTs) were grown in the C$_{60}$-pyridine solution or C$_{60}$-NMP solution which was exposed to the visible light. The type of solvents plays a critical role in the formation of the final structure of C$_{60}$ FNFs.

Self-assembled by zero dimensional fullerenes, FNFs, who maintain the conjugated π-electron structure of fullerene and features of one dimensional materials, show promising novel optoelectronic and magnetic properties.

---

[1] E-mail address: piao@qust.edu.cn

In: Chemistry Research Summaries Volume 12
Editor: Lucille Monaco Cacioppo

ISBN: 978-1-61668-757-1
© 2014 Nova Science Publishers, Inc.

Chapter 62

RADIATION INDUCED PHENOMENA IN FULLERENES

G. Ya. Gerasimov

Institute of Mechanics, Moscow State University,
Moscow, Russia

RESEARCH SUMMARY

This chapter gives an analysis of various radiation effects in fullerenes caused by their interaction with energetic particles (electrons or ions). The most important of them that lead to transformation of the fullerene structure are displacement of carbon atoms from fullerene surface, breakage of interatomic bonds or their cross-linking and collective electronic excitation of fullerene cage. These effects determine limits of stability and possible mechanisms of fullerene-based structures destruction and modification. The main mechanism of fullerene molecule destruction under action of high-energy electron beam at energies more than 100 keV is elastic collisions of electrons with atoms of the carbon cage, which leads to knock-on displacement of carbon atoms from the cage surface. A theoretical study of this process was performed using an analytical expression for the cross-section for scattering of relativistic electrons by carbon atoms, as well as the threshold energy of atom displacement from the fullerene surface obtained by the molecular dynamic method.

In: Chemistry Research Summaries Volume 12
Editor: Lucille Monaco Cacioppo

ISBN: 978-1-61668-757-1
© 2014 Nova Science Publishers, Inc.

Chapter 63

Fabrication and Characterization of Phthalocyanine/C_{60}-Based Solar Cells with Diamond Nanoclusters

Takeo Oku[1,], Akihiko Nagata[1], Akihiro Takeda[1], Akira Minowa[1], Atsushi Suzuki[1], Kenji Kikuchi[1], Yasuhiro Yamasaki[2] and Eiji Ōsawa[3]*

[1]Department of Materials Science, The University of Shiga Prefecture,
Hikone, Shiga, Japan
[2]Orient Chemical Industries Co., Ltd., Department of New Business,
Neyagawa, Osaka, Japan
[3]NanoCarbon Research Institute, Ltd., Nagano, Japan

Research Summary

C_{60}/phthalocyanine-based bulk heterojunction and heterojunction solar cells were fabricated, and the electronic and optical properties were investigated. Fullerene (C_{60}) and fullerenol ($C_{60}(OH)_{10-12}$) were used as n-type semiconductors, and diamond nanoparticles, metal phthalocyanine derivative and μ-oxo-bridged gallium phthalocyanine dimer were used as p-type semiconductors. The nanostructures of the solar cells were investigated by transmission electron microscopy and X-ray diffraction, and the electronic property was discussed. Electronic structures of the molecules were investigated by molecular orbital calculation, and energy levels of the solar cells were discussed.

---

* E-mail address: oku@mat.usp.ac.jp

In: Chemistry Research Summaries Volume 12
Editor: Lucille Monaco Cacioppo

ISBN: 978-1-61668-757-1
© 2014 Nova Science Publishers, Inc.

Chapter 64

SURFACE CHEMICAL MODIFICATION OF FULLERENE BASED COLLOIDS

Z. Marković, S. Jovanović and B. Todorović Marković[1]
Vinča Institute of Nuclear Sciences, University of Belgrade, Belgrade, Serbia

RESEARCH SUMMARY

In this chapter, comparative analysis of the properties of fullerene based colloids synthesized by two different methods has been presented. Fullerene based colloids have been synthesized by solvent exchange method and mechanochemical treatment. During synthesis by solvent exchange method, tetrahydrofuran (THF) was used as a solvent. For mechanochemical treatment of fullerene different encapsulating agents have been used: THF/ETOH, sodium dodecyl sulfate (SDS), sodium dodecylbenzene sulfonate (SDBS) and ethylene vinyl acetate-ethylene vinyl versatate (EVA-EVV), respectively. The properties of prepared colloids have been investigated by different techniques: atomic force microscopy, UV/Vis and Fourier transform infrared (FTIR) spectroscopy. By means of atomic force microscopy size and shape of fullerene nanoparticles have been investigated. FTIR measurements for fullerene colloids synthesized by solvent exchange method have shown the bonding among THF molecules and fullerene nanocrystals. As for fullerene based colloids prepared by mechanochemical treatment FTIR analyses has shown the presence of pure C_{60} after surface functionalization.

---

[1] E-mail address: email.biljatod@vinca.rs

In: Chemistry Research Summaries Volume 12
Editor: Lucille Monaco Cacioppo
ISBN: 978-1-61668-757-1
© 2014 Nova Science Publishers, Inc.

Chapter 65

COMPUTATIONAL DESIGN OF NEW ORGANIC MATERIALS: PROPERTIES AND UTILITY OF METHYLENE-BRIDGED FULLERENES C60

Ken Tokunaga[1]

Division of Liberal Arts, Kogakuin University,
Tokyo, Japan

RESEARCH SUMMARY

Fullerene C_{60} and its derivatives have recently been found to be very useful as organic semiconductors for organic devices such as the organic field-effect transistor (OFET). In this chapter, effect of methylene-bridging on carrier transport properties of C_{60} is theoretically estimated and is systematically discussed using the density functional theory (DFT) calculation, by taking methylene-bridged fullerene C_{60} CX_2 (X=H, halogen, R, R-COOH, and R-SH, where R is alkyl chain) as examples. Based on the Marcus theory, carrier transport properties are related to the reorganization energy. Hole-transport property of methylene-bridged C_{60} is strongly dependent on the kind (chemical properties) of *X*. On the other hand, electron-transport property of C_{60} is little influenced by the methylene bridging. These results are discussed from viewpoints of geometric and electronic structures. It is found that the values of reorganization energies are closely related to the change in bridged C• • •C distance upon the carrier injection. Strong anti-bonding character of frontier orbitals around bridged C atoms results in large reorganization energy and slow carrier transport. From these analyses, specific guidelines for efficient design of useful organic semiconductors are proposed.

---

[1] E-mail address: tokunaga@cc.kogakuin.ac.jp

In: Chemistry Research Summaries Volume 12   ISBN: 978-1-61668-757-1
Editor: Lucille Monaco Cacioppo   © 2014 Nova Science Publishers, Inc.

Chapter 66

THE ROLE OF HYDROGEN PEROXIDE ON ADVANCED OXIDATION PROCESSES OF WATER CONTAMINANTS AT AMBIENT CONDITIONS

Fernando J. Beltrán, Almudena Aguinaco and Ana Rey
Departamento de Ingeniería Química y Química Física,
Universidad de Extremadura, Badajoz, Spain

RESEARCH SUMMARY

Hydrogen peroxide together to chlorine, chlorine dioxide, permanganate and ozone are one of the important oxidants used in water treatment. Although kinetics of hydrogen peroxide reactions with water pollutants, especially organic pollutants, is relatively low, hydrogen peroxide presents a high capacity to be combined with other oxidants and agents (catalysts or radiation) to initiate radical chain mechanisms that lead to the formation of hydroxyl radicals. These processes, named as advanced oxidation processes, are the main route to total elimination of pollutants that otherwise will remain in water or in another phase. Advanced oxidation processes involving hydrogen peroxide can be classified as ambient conditions (pressure and temperature) or wet oxidation conditions (high pressure and temperature) processes. This chapter will deal with the ambient conditions hydrogen peroxide advanced oxidation processes (H_2O_2AOP) which are suitable for both surface water or low concentrated wastewater treatment. H_2O_2AOP can also be classified as those where the oxidant is generated in situ (single ozonation, catalytic oxidation, etc.) and other where hydrogen peroxide is added to the system (Fenton, ozone-peroxide, hydrogen peroxide photolysis, etc.). Main mechanisms of reactions, kinetics and review of recent literature on these H_2O_2AOP for the treatment of water contaminants will be presented in the chapter.

In: Chemistry Research Summaries Volume 12
Editor: Lucille Monaco Cacioppo

ISBN: 978-1-61668-757-1
© 2014 Nova Science Publishers, Inc.

Chapter 67

Electrochemical Approach to Quantify Cellular Hydrogen Peroxide and Monitor Its Release Process from Living Cells

Ping Wu, Hui Zhang and Chenxin Cai

Jiangsu Key Laboratory of New Power Batteries,
College of Chemistry and Materials Science, Nanjing Normal University, China

RESEARCH SUMMARY

Hydrogen peroxide (H_2O_2) is one of significant representative of reactive oxygen species (ROS), it can express diverse physiological and pathological consequences within living systems in a concentration-dependent manner. At its low concentration, H_2O_2 functions as the second messenger for several growth factors, cytokines, and signal transduction. Whereas high concentration of H_2O_2 is a source of oxidative damage to cellular equilibrium leading to aging, Alzheimer's and related neurodegenerative diseases, cardiovascular disorders, even cancer. This chapter introduces the methods to detect cellular H_2O_2, including colorimetry, electrochemical methods, chemiluminescence, fluorescence, and electron spin resonance, etc., and mainly describes the electrochemical approach to quantify the level of H_2O_2 in various cell lines and monitor the release process of H_2O_2 from the living cells. Electrochemical detection approaches depicted in this chapter are based on electrochemical reduction of H_2O_2 catalyzed by enzymes (including proteins) and nanomaterials. Horseradish peroxidase (HRP), and hemoglobin (Hb) were selected as model enzyme and protein, nitrogen-doped graphene (N-graphene) was chosen as a representative of nanomaterials to catalyze H_2O_2. The preparation, immoblization, characterization, and application of the above mentioned catalysts to detect cellular H_2O_2, to study kinetics on the exocytotic process, and to evaluate the whole efficiency of the process in real-time are introduced. These results presented in this chapter open a new way for quantification cellular H_2O_2 level and also develop a new platform for a reliable collection of kinetic information on cellular H_2O_2 release, which could be potentially useful in study of downstream biological effects in physiology and pathology.

In: Chemistry Research Summaries Volume 12
Editor: Lucille Monaco Cacioppo

ISBN: 978-1-61668-757-1
© 2014 Nova Science Publishers, Inc.

Chapter 68

HYDROGEN PEROXIDE: ROLE IN INFLAMMATION

Stefania Marzocco, Giuseppe Bianco and Giuseppina Autore

Department of Pharmaceutical and Biomedical Sciences, University of Salerno,
Fisciano, SA, Italy

RESEARCH SUMMARY

Hydrogen peroxide (H_2O_2) is an highly reactive compound produced by cells after secondary reactions as result of the leakage of electrons from the electron transport chain in mitochondria or as a consequence of other enzymatic reactions.

H_2O_2 is able to oxidize and thereby to induce damage in numerous cellular constituents. Over the last decade it has become accepted that H_2O_2 serves important biological roles outside of its capacity to cause oxidative damage. The main factor which determines H_2O_2 effects is its own level associated to the activation of different redox-sensitive transcription factors and to distinct biological responses. Once accumulates in cells, H_2O_2 can, for example, modify proteins and the underlining mechanisms involved attracting great interest at the moment. One of the main proteins target for H_2O_2 is the thiol group of the amino acid cysteine in protein regulating many cell responses (e.g., phosphatases and transcription factors).

Inflammation is a crucial function of the innate immune system that protects host tissues against dangerous insults that are detrimental to tissue homeostasis, including wound damage and pathogen invasion. During the course of inflammatory processes, H_2O_2 may be generated in large amounts. This occurrence may be due to the activation of mast cells, macrophages, eosinophils, and neutrophils, which generate superoxide radical ($O_2^{.-}$), predominantly via NADPH oxidase (NOX). Superoxide dismutase (SOD) rapidly converts $O_2^{.-}$ into H_2O_2 which can easily penetrate the membranes of surrounding cells. There is no known receptor for H_2O_2, but potentially H_2O_2 gradients might be "read" via intracellular sensors such as phosphatases that subsequently regulate the chemotactic response. Alternatively, there may be other extracellular (or intracellular) substrates that H_2O_2 modifies in some way to convert them into chemotactic factors or other modulators of cell motility. Several observations suggest that H_2O_2 acts as a common second messenger following cellular exposure to agents that induce inflammatory response. Interactions between H_2O_2 and inflammatory mediator (e.g., NF-κB) might be a component of the intracellular signalling process that leads to inflammation. Treatment with H_2O_2 directly activates NF-κB in some cells, and over expression of SOD, enhances the tumor necrosis factor-α induced activation of NF-κB. In this context H_2O_2 represent a messenger able to alter redox homeostasis contributing, at several levels, to inflammatory-related disease. Despite H_2O_2 is not an inherently reactive compound it can be also converted into highly reactive and deleterious products killing cells. This is a non-specific process direct to pathogens but it can induce damage also to the human body.

Here we describe the role of H_2O_2 in cellular signalling focusing our attention on H_2O_2 role in inflammation. Moreover we also examine the H_2O_2 signalling in some cardiovascular, renal and pulmonary inflammatory-based disease.

In: Chemistry Research Summaries Volume 12   ISBN: 978-1-61668-757-1
Editor: Lucille Monaco Cacioppo   © 2014 Nova Science Publishers, Inc.

Chapter 69

HYDROGEN PEROXIDE DEPLETES PHOSPHATIDYLINOSITOL-3-PHOSPHATE FROM ENDOSOMES IN A P38 MAPK-DEPENDENT MANNER AND PERTURBS ENDOCYTIC TRANSPORT AND SIGNAL TRANSDUCTION IN PATHOGENIC CELLS

Masayuki Murata and Fumi Kano

Department of Life Sciences, Graduate School of Arts and Sciences,
The University of Tokyo, Tokyo, Japan

RESEARCH SUMMARY

Hydrogen peroxide (H_2O_2) has gained much attention not only as a stressor that oxidizes components of the cell but also as signaling molecule in physiological processes. On the minus side, elevation of reactive oxygen species (ROS) including H_2O_2 causes oxidative stress, and is reported to be involved in many diseases, such as diabetes, atherosclerosis, Parkinson's disease, and Alzheimer's disease. On the plus side, H_2O_2 is produced when cells respond to various stimuli, and mediates downstream signals. Recently, we found that H_2O_2 treatment depleted HeLa cell endosomes of phosphatidylinositol-3-phosphate (PI3P). To quantify and visualize the intracellular localization of PI3P we have developed a novel analytical method that employs a semi-intact cell system, a permeabilized cell that enables the addition of various exogenous molecules into the cells, and protein probe for PI3P, GST-2xFYVE protein. Using this method, we found that H_2O_2 decreased the amount of PI3P in endosomes in a manner dependent upon p38 MAPK, a kinase that is activated during oxidative stress or pathogenic conditions. In addition, H_2O_2 treatment delayed vesicular transport in a broad range of endocytic pathways: the lysosomal degradation of EGFR, the retrograde transport of cholera toxin from the plasma membrane to the *trans*-Golgi network (TGN), and the uptake and recycling of transferrin.

The physiological role of PI3P in endosomes has received a lot of attention with respect to endocytosis and signal transduction via endosomes. For example, PI3P in the endosomal membrane appears to act as a microdomain for the recruitment of various proteins that contain a PI3P-binding (FYVE) domain. Interestingly, FYVE-containing proteins are involved not only in the regulation of endosomal processing but also in signal transduction via endosomes.

In this chapter, we demonstrate the effect of H_2O_2 on early endocytic pathways and discuss the utility of H_2O_2 as a useful oxidative stressor to investigate various intracellular events under pathological conditions.

In: Chemistry Research Summaries Volume 12   ISBN: 978-1-61668-757-1
Editor: Lucille Monaco Cacioppo   © 2014 Nova Science Publishers, Inc.

Chapter 70

USES OF HYDROGEN PEROXIDE IN AQUACULTURE

Gemma Giménez Papiol[1] and Ana Roque[2]*
[1]Cawthron Institute, Nelson, New Zealand
[2]IRTA Sant Carles de la Ràpita,
Institut de Recerca i Tecnologia Agroalimentàries, Barcelona, Spain

RESEARCH SUMMARY

In this chapter we revise the uses of hydrogen peroxide in aquaculture. At the beginning, hydrogen peroxide was used mainly as a treatment against ectoparasites of adult fish, such as sea lice (*Lepeophtherius salmonis*), or against the microbiota of fish eggs, mainly fungi in freshwater species.

Later, it became of interest for microbial control purposes rather than chlorine or antibiotics due to its relatively lower toxicity. Although it is one of the most powerful known oxidizers, it is easily decomposed in a water solution, particularly in the presence of organic matter, light and turbulence (all conditions easily met in aquaculture systems), leaving no toxic products. The spectrum of species and live stages has also increased; hydrogen peroxide has been tested on rotifers, crustacea, bivalves and fish, and on eggs, larvae, juveniles and adults.

Recently, issues concerning its impact on the aquaculture system (i.e., biofilters of the recirculation system), on the environment and on animal welfare of cultured species have risen.

* Correspondence: G. Giménez-Papiol, Cawthron Institute, 98 Halifax Street East, Private Bag 2, Nelson 7042, New Zealand. E-mail: Gemma.GimenezPapiol@cawthron.org.nz

In: Chemistry Research Summaries Volume 12   ISBN: 978-1-61668-757-1
Editor: Lucille Monaco Cacioppo   © 2014 Nova Science Publishers, Inc.

Chapter 71

FUNCTIONS OF HYDROGEN PEROXIDE IN REGULATING FUNGAL VIABILITY AND PATHOGENICITY

Shiping Tian, Guozheng Qin, Boqiang Li and Zhang Zhanquan
Key Laboratory of Plant Resources, Institute of Botany,
Chinese Academy of Sciences, Beijing, China

RESEARCH SUMMARY

As known as well, the active oxygen species hydrogen peroxide (H_2O_2) has been proven to play critical roles in various cellular activities, including the direct cause of membrane damage, the component of structural defense, the signal molecule operating within the challenged cell and the antimicrobial compound because of H_2O_2 acting as a signal molecule in the induction of systemic acquired resistance.

In addition, H_2O_2 is relatively stable, can diffuse freely throughout the cell, and has a similarly low reactivity toward biological molecules. In this review, we mainly summarize the functions of hydrogen peroxide in regulating the viability of antagonistic yeasts and the pathogenicity of fungal pathogens, as well as the molecular targets of hydrogen peroxide in fungal cells.

In: Chemistry Research Summaries Volume 12   ISBN: 978-1-61668-757-1
Editor: Lucille Monaco Cacioppo   © 2014 Nova Science Publishers, Inc.

Chapter 72

ELECTROCHEMICAL CHARACTERIZATION OF O_2 METABOLISM IN ISOLATED MITOCHONDRIA REVEALED MASSIVE PRODUCTION OF H_2O_2 UPON ATP SYNTHASE ACTIVATION

Raluca Marcu[1,], Stefania Rapino[1], Francesco Paolucci[2] and Marco Giorgio[1]*

[1]European Institute of Oncology, Department of Experimental Oncology, Milan, Italy
[2]University of Bologna, Department of Chemistry "G. Ciamician," Bologna, Italy

RESEARCH SUMMARY

The mitochondrial reactive oxygen species (ROS) production is a crucial issue that has been involved in a variety of physio-pathological processes and aging. However, at the present measurements of mitochondrial ROS production is controversial. Indeed, the available tools are poorly specific and not direct.

Now taking advantage of the progress in microelectrode production it has been possible to approach the specific and direct measurement of O_2 species in a suspension of isolated mitochondria.

Such electrochemical determinations confirm active H_2O_2 release by mitochondria above the scavenging activity and reveal a significant role of ATP synthase activation in the control of mitochondrial ROS production.

These findings offer a new explanation for the effects of mitochondrial respiration on oxidative stress. Regardless the damaging effect of ROS that has been already associated to intense mitochondrial work during exercise in muscle for example, H_2O_2 spikes may represent specific cellular signal. The crosstalk between the mitochondrion and the cell is indeed an emergent issue. About this argument our observation discloses a novel basic mechanism of mitochondrial ROS production and highlights the involvement of intracellular redox balance on health.

---

* Authors contact info: marco.giorgio@ifom-ieo-campus.it ; Tel: +39-02-94375040; Fax +39-02-94375990.

In: Chemistry Research Summaries Volume 12   ISBN: 978-1-61668-757-1
Editor: Lucille Monaco Cacioppo   © 2014 Nova Science Publishers, Inc.

Chapter 73

DETERMINATION OF SCAVENGING CAPACITY AGAINST HYDROGEN PEROXIDE: RECENT TRENDS ON CHEMICAL METHODS

Marcela A. Segundo, Carla Castro, Luís M. Magalhães and Salette Reis*

REQUIMTE, Department of Chemical Sciences,
Faculty of Pharmacy, University of Porto, Porto, Portugal

RESEARCH SUMMARY

Hydrogen peroxide is one of the most important reactive oxygen species and it has gained an enormous attention due to its high permeability within cell and across cellular membranes, as an in vivo precursor of strong oxidants (namely hydroxyl radical and hypochlorous acid) and due to its implication in the generation of superoxide radical anion. Therefore, the development of reliable analytical methods to determine the scavenging capacity against hydrogen peroxide has been a topic of increased interest within pharmaceutical and biomedical area. Currently, several methods are available for performing the determination of scavenging capacity against hydrogen peroxide using UV–vis spectrophotometry, fluorescence and chemiluminescence as detection systems. In this chapter, a critical review of these methods will be undertaken, by comparing the figures of merit and limitations provided by some of the most applied methods (measurement of intrinsic absorption of H_2O_2 in UV region, fluorimetric assays based in scopoletin and homovanillic acid, chemiluminescence quenching of luminol and lucigenin, among others). Moreover, special emphasis will be given to methods developed in the last three years, based on automatic systems and nanotechnology breakthroughs.

---

* Corresponding author. Phone +351 220428676; fax +351 226093483, E-mail: msegundo@ff.up.pt.

In: Chemistry Research Summaries Volume 12
Editor: Lucille Monaco Cacioppo

ISBN: 978-1-61668-757-1
© 2014 Nova Science Publishers, Inc.

Chapter 74

HYDROGEN PEROXIDE: A VERSATILE AND ENVIRONMENTALLY BENIGN OXIDANT OF NATURAL OLEFINS ABLE WITH DIFFERENT CATALYSTS

*Ligia Mendonça Maria Vieira[1], Milene Lopes da Silva[1] and Márcio José da Silva[1]**

[1]Federal University of Viçosa, Chemistry Department,
Viçosa, Minas Gerais, Brazil

RESEARCH SUMMARY

This chapter summarizes our recent developments for H_2O_2 based green oxidation reactions, using two different transition metal catalysts: palladium and cobalt. Results obtained from the oxidation of the natural olefins using as oxidant the hydrogen peroxide and as catalysts palladium and cobalt chlorides are presented and discussed in mechanistic terms. Monoterpenes are abundant and renewable raw materials and when converted into oxygenates products are valuable ingredient for fragrance, agrochemicals and pharmaceutical industries. Camphene, β-pinene and 3-carene are monoterpenes of high natural occurrence, which oxygenated derivates, are highly attractive for fine chemical and fragrances industry and for these reasons were the selected substrates. The different aspects involved in the oxidation of these substrates in presence of two different catalysts were assessed. Palladium(II)-catalyzed oxidation reactions proceeds via two electrons intermediates (heterolytic oxidation); conversely, Cobalt(II)-catalyzed oxidation reactions occurs via one electrons intermediates (homolytic oxidation). In all most of the catalytic reactions, high conversion substrates were achieved. Moreover, the selectivity of the oxidation products can be controlled by molar ratio substrate:oxidant and by temperature of reaction. Hydrogen peroxide, an environmentally benign reactant, regardless catalyst employed was an efficient oxidant in the conversion of monoterpenes into valuable oxygenates derivates.

---

* Email: silvamj2003@ufv.br

In: Chemistry Research Summaries Volume 12
Editor: Lucille Monaco Cacioppo

ISBN: 978-1-61668-757-1
© 2014 Nova Science Publishers, Inc.

Chapter 75

ENVIRONMENTAL FATE OF POLYCYCLIC AROMATIC HYDROCARBONS EMITTED FROM INDOOR BURNING OF FUEL BIOMASS IN POORLY VENTILATED HOUSEHOLDS: A CASE STUDY IN THE TRADITIONAL RURAL HOUSEHOLDS IN WESTERN KENYA

Fred Ayodi Lisouza[1]*, P. Okinda Owuor[1]
and Joseph O. Lalah[2]

[1]Department of Chemistry, Maseno University, Kenya
[2]Department of Chemical Science and Technology,
Kenya Polytechnic University College, Kenya

RESEARCH SUMMARY

Anthropogenic sources of polycyclic aromatic hydrocarbons (PAHs) to the environment are more abundant than natural sources. However, information on the environmental fate of PAHs from point sources is scarce. This chapter gives a survey of the characterization, levels, and the environmental fate of PAHs resulting from indoor biomass burning inside poorly ventilated households. It gives original research findings as well as a critical review of other research findings published on this subject area. Western Kenya has prevalence of grass-roofed traditional houses, where cooking is done in open fire places using various biomass types, which leads to accumulation of soot under the roofs. PAHs result from incomplete combustion of organic compounds and are emitted in gaseous phase, which may adsorb on to soot particles, or particulate phase. Exposure to mixtures of PAHs increases incidences of cancer in human populations. The high indoor temperatures probably cause volatilisation of the adsorbed PAHs, leading to higher continuous human exposure to PAHs. Data indicate that cancer cases are rampant in the region, yet no studies had been done to show potential causes of these cancers. The objective of this study was to extract, characterize and quantify the

* E-mail: lisouzafred@yahoo.com, Tel: +254722612153

levels of PAHs on soot deposits in grass-roofed houses in Western Kenya and to determine the variations in concentration of PAHs on the soot deposits with biomass type used and house age, and hence determine if the patterns of PAHs accumulation on the soot deposits significantly vary with the biomass fuel type. The houses were classified according to the predominant biomass fuel source and house age (0-5, 5-10, >10 years). The study design was factorial two, laid out in randomised complete block arrangements with fuel source as the main factor and house age as the second factor. The soot samples, collected from four houses in each sampling unit, were extracted by Soxhlet using dichloromethane, cleaned on silica gel column and analyzed by gas chromatography using open tubular capillary columns with flame ionization detector. Identification of PAHs was based on retention times of authentic standards and verified by gas chromatographic-mass spectral analysis. Quantification was based on peak area responses using the internal standard method and concentrations corrected for recovery. Separation of means and analysis of variance was done using a factorial two in randomized complete block design model. The PAHs levels have been reported to significantly ($P \leq 0.05$) vary with predominant fuel source in the order: Dung $\geq$ perennial indigenous trees $\geq$ exotic trees $\geq$ shrubs and crop residues. This study reveals that PAHs emitted during indoor biomass burning significantly accumulate ($P \leq 0.05$) on soot deposits under the roofs with time. The results of this study further show that the accumulation patterns of some PAHs vary significantly ($P \leq 0.05$) with variation in biomass type used. These findings indicate that the patterns of accumulation of the PAHs from biomass fuel combustion are not homogenous across all the biomass types under study.

In: Chemistry Research Summaries Volume 12   ISBN: 978-1-61668-757-1
Editor: Lucille Monaco Cacioppo   © 2014 Nova Science Publishers, Inc.

Chapter 76

POLYCYCLIC AROMATIC HYDROCARBONS IN FOODS AND HERBAL MEDICINES: ANALYSIS AND OCCURRENCE

Hiroyuki Kataoka and Atsushi Ishizaki
School of Pharmacy, Shujitsu University, Nishigawara, Okayama, Japan

RESEARCH SUMMARY

Polycyclic aromatic hydrocarbons (PAHs) are a group of about 10,000 different compounds containing two or more fused aromatic rings made of carbon and hydrogen atoms. Some PAHs are highly carcinogenic and/or genotoxic in laboratory animals and have been implicated in breast, lung, and colon cancers in humans. PAHs are ubiquitous environmental pollutants, resulting from the incomplete combustion or pyrolysis of organic matter during industrial processing and various human activities. Environmental PAHs can be introduced into the food chain by both plants and animals. Furthermore, food can become contaminated during thermal treatments that occur in processes of food preparation and manufacture (e.g., heating, drying and smoking processes), by contact with packaging materials and by certain cooking methods (e.g., grilling, roasting, baking, and frying processes). Smoke flavoring products, utilized to improve organoleptic characteristics in the food industry and produced from smoke condensates, are another significant source of PAHs in foods. Among the foods containing PAHs at μg/kg or ng/L concentrations are edible oils, fruits, vegetables, coffee, tea, beverages, seafood, smoked fish, smoked meat, smoked cheese, milk, honey, dried foods, cooked foods, and food supplements. Furthermore, many herbal medicines are dried using combustion gases and are in direct contact with PAHs, leading to their accumulation in these products. Although exposure to PAHs has become a significant public health problem, the multiple sources of human exposure make it difficult to assess the contribution due to intake of single foods and herbal medicines. In view of the recognized adverse effects of PAHs and the need for regulatory control, monitoring of their levels in foods and herbal products is important in evaluating the risks associated with human consumption. In this chapter, we review advances in sample preparation and analysis of PAHs, and their sources and occurrence in foods and herbal medicines.

In: Chemistry Research Summaries Volume 12
Editor: Lucille Monaco Cacioppo

ISBN: 978-1-61668-757-1
© 2014 Nova Science Publishers, Inc.

Chapter 77

BIOMONITORING OF POLYCYCLIC AROMATIC HYDROCARBONS BY PINE NEEDLES – LEVELS AND TRENDS IN SOUTHERN EUROPE

Nuno Ratola[1,2,*], José Manuel Amigo[3], Silvia Lacorte[4],
Damià Barceló[4,5], Elefteria Psillakis[6] and Arminda Alves[1]

[1]LEPAE, Department of Chemical Engineering, Faculty of Engineering,
University of Porto, Porto, Portugal
[2]Physics of the Earth, University of Murcia, Edificio CIOyN,
Campus de Espinardo, Murcia, Spain
[3]Department of Food Science, Quality and Technology, Faculty of Life Sciences,
University of Copenhagen, Frederiksberg C, Denmark
[4]Department of Environmental Chemistry, IDAEA-CSIC, Barcelona, Spain
[5]Catalan Institute for Water Research (ICRA), Edifici H2O,
Parc Científic i Tecnologíc de la Universitat de Girona, Girona, Spain
[6]Department of Environmental Engineering, Technical University
of Crete, Polytechneioupolis, Chania, Greece

RESEARCH SUMMARY

Polycyclic aromatic hydrocarbons (PAHs) are widespread carcinogenic and mutagenic contaminants with natural and anthropogenic sources mainly associated to combustion processes. The monitoring of these types of semi-volatile organic pollutants is a crucial step to assess their environmental exposure to organisms. Although in general this task is performed directly in their own habitat, biomonitoring offers the possibility to estimate the multi-route uptake of contaminants. Vegetation has been used for some time due to its worldwide presence, adequate uptake conditions and low availability costs. These valuable matrices allow the passive sampling of a wide range of compounds, mainly airborne. PAHs are no exception since their hydrophobic and lipophylic nature make them prone to partition

* E-mail: nrneto@fe.up.pt.

into the waxy layers of plants and trees (mostly on the leaves) or, in the case of the heavier particle-bound PAHs, to be deposited in the surface.

However, handling plant matrices is a complex mission to accomplish, in particular the separation of the target compounds from their lipidic structure. This led to the development of multiresidue extraction methods in the past two decades, in a demand for reliable extraction and clean-up procedures and increasingly lower limits of detection associated with enhanced chromatographic resolution.

The main objective of this chapter is to present the concentrations, aromatic ring patterns and possible sources of 16 PAHs extracted from pine needles in three different countries from the South of Europe (Portugal, Spain and Greece) and try to point out potential similarities and differences in their behaviour, separating urban and non-urban areas. A total of 90 sampling sites (29 in Portugal, 34 in Spain and 27 in Greece) were selected in urban, industrial, rural and remote areas. The use of chemometric methods (namely principal component analysis - PCA) was of significant importance in the analysis and interpretation of the large environmental biomonitoring dataset produced.

The PAH levels were, in general, higher in Greece, followed by Portugal and Spain, with predominance of 3- and 4-ring PAHs. Some visible differences were found in the aromatic ring patterns (and possibly in the sources) between urban and non-urban sites in the three countries. PCA further confirmed these trends, clearly separating the urban and the non-urban sites and all three countries, which suggests that the sources of contamination vary in each case and demonstrates the suitability of pine needles for trans-boundary biomonitoring of atmospheric PAHs.

In: Chemistry Research Summaries Volume 12
Editor: Lucille Monaco Cacioppo

ISBN: 978-1-61668-757-1
© 2014 Nova Science Publishers, Inc.

Chapter 78

INVESTIGATION ON BIODEGRADATION OF A MODEL POLYCYCLIC AROMATIC HYDROCARBONS (PAHS) COMPOUND - ANTHRACENE (ANT) - BY *FUSARIUM SOLANI* MAS2 ISOLATED FROM MANGROVE SEDIMENT

Yi-Rui Wu[1,2,], Zhu-Hua Luo[3] and L. L. P. Vrijmoed[2]*
[1]Department of Civil and Environmental Engineering,
Faculty of Engineering, National University of Singapore, Singapore
[2]Department of Biology and Chemistry, City University of Hong Kong,
Kowloon, Hong Kong SAR, P. R. China
[3]Key Laboratory of Marine Biogenetic Resources, Third Institute
of Oceanography, State Oceanic Administration, Xiamen, P. R. China

RESEARCH SUMMARY

Polycyclic aromatic hydrocarbons (PAHs) are a class of important environmental pollutants that usually occured during the uncompleted combustion process. They are of major concern due to their widespread in our surroundings, persistence, toxicity and especially the carcinogenic property. Microbial biodegradation is one of the most important natural processes which can influence the fate of pollutants in both terrestrial and aquatic environment. Mangroves and wetlands usually serve as sinks of different kinds of environmental pollutants, which lead to the possibility of the occurrence of a diversity of microbes with degradative capabilities.

Actually, bacterial degradation of PAHs is well documented, however, little information is available on the biodegradation on PAHs by mangrove sediment fungi. The investigation aims to isolate PAHs-degrading fungal species from mangrove sediment, to explore the

---

* Corresponding Author: Dr. Yi-Rui WU. Tel: +65 93759745; Email: oxwyr@tom.com.

degradative pathways, and to further analyze the related key enzyme (e.g., laccase) with anthracene (ANT) as the model PAHs.

In this study, one ANT-degrading fungus, namely as MAS2, was isolated from the PAHs-contaminated mangrove sediment collected from Ma Wan in Hong Kong by the enrichment with ANT as the sole carbon source, and identified as *Fusarium solani* based on the morphology and molecular typing using 18S rDNA sequence. Analysis on the degradative percentage demonstrated that *F. solani* MAS2 could remove 20 mg l^{-1} of ANT during the 40 days of incubation.

Investigation by solid phase microextraction (SPME) combined with gas chromatography equipped with mass spectrometry (GC/MS) indicated that strain MAS2 performed the traditional pathway by tranformaing ANT into phthalic acid through its quinone molecule (9,10-anthracenedione). During the degradation of ANT by *F. solani* MAS2, laccase was detected as the important lignin-degradation related enzyme involved in the biodegradation of PAHs by fungi. The purification and characterization of laccase were also carried out to suggest the novelty of this enzyme as well as its important role in ANT degrdation.

In: Chemistry Research Summaries Volume 12
Editor: Lucille Monaco Cacioppo

ISBN: 978-1-61668-757-1
© 2014 Nova Science Publishers, Inc.

Chapter 79

SOURCES, DISTRIBUTIONS AND FORENSIC APPLICATIONS OF POLYCYCLIC AROMATIC HYDROCARBONS (PAHS) IN THE NIGER DELTA REGION OF NIGERIA: AN OVERVIEW

B. O. Ekpo[1,*], E. P. Fubara[2] and V. E. Etuk[3]

[1]Environmental and Petroleum Geochemistry Research Group (EPGRG),
Department of Pure and Applied Chemistry,
University of Calabar, Calabar, C. R. State, Nigeria
[2]Department of Chemistry, Rivers State University of Education,
Port Harcourt, Nigeria
[3]Department of Chemical Engineering,
University of Uyo, Akwa Ibom State, Nigeria

RESEARCH SUMMARY

Rapid developments in industrial and agricultural activities, urbanization and the use of chemicals have been known to have serious negative environmental implications globally. This is literally the situation with the Niger Delta region of Nigeria since the discovery of oil in Oloibiri in the present-day Bayelsa State in 1956. This Chapter summarizes published scientific data on polycyclic aromatic hydrocarbons (PAHs) in the environment of the Niger Delta region. It provides an overview on the levels of PAHs, their distributions and sources in soils, water, estuarine sediments, marine organisms, and application in environmental forensics. The data preliminarily reveal the state of contamination/pollution in this region and provide an insight into the fate of PAHs in a typical tropical area, where researches on environmental samples are mostly limited to sediments, soils and biota.

---

* Corresponding Author: Phone: +234 08037183898; E-mail: baekpo@yahoo.com.

In: Chemistry Research Summaries Volume 12   ISBN: 978-1-61668-757-1
Editor: Lucille Monaco Cacioppo   © 2014 Nova Science Publishers, Inc.

Chapter 80

THERMODYNAMICS AND PHASE BEHAVIOR OF POLYCYCLIC AROMATIC HYDROCARBON MIXTURES

James W. Rice[,1], Jinxia Fu[2] and Eric M. Suuberg[1]*

[1]Brown University School of Engineering, Providence, Rhode Island, US
[2]Brown University Department of Chemistry, Providence, Rhode Island, US

RESEARCH SUMMARY

PAHs are quite regularly found in mixtures of similarly structured compounds and there is surprisingly little in the way of reliable phase behavior information on PAH mixtures in the literature. The research conducted in this laboratory has, for some time, been motivated by this deficiency and aimed at a thorough investigation of the thermodynamics and phase behavior of PAH mixtures. Binary PAH mixtures examined here, i.e., anthracene + pyrene and anthracene + benzo[a]pyrene, were highly non-ideal. Formation of eutectic phases, azeotropy, and accommodation of low-level impurities were observed in both cases. This behavior has been attributed to formation of cluster-like entities that define the thermodynamics and associated phase behavior of the mixtures. This non-ideal behavior observed here for few-component mixtures is general. The important message is that PAH mixtures, and potentially other mixtures with a finite number of agents, may be surprising non-ideal. Beyond these few component mixtures, PAH tars form as the number of mixture components increases. Tarlike behavior was observed and reported for 5- and 6- component PAH mixtures. Results suggested that the vapor pressure of these tarlike mixtures could be predicted by ideal mixture theory, i.e., Raoult's law. Despite this transition to a seemingly more environmentally relevant mixture, the phase behavior of such "tars" might become complicated as components are lost via evaporation or other transport processes.

In: Chemistry Research Summaries Volume 12
Editor: Lucille Monaco Cacioppo

ISBN: 978-1-61668-757-1
© 2014 Nova Science Publishers, Inc.

Chapter 81

OCCURRENCE OF POLYCYCLIC AROMATIC HYDROCARBONS IN CEPHALOPODS

Simone Morais[1]*, Filipa Gomes[1], Maria João Ramalhosa[1],
Cristina Delerue-Matos[1] and Maria Beatriz Prior Pinto Oliveira[2]#

[1]REQUIMTE, Instituto Superior de Engenharia do Porto, Portugal
[2]REQUIMTE, Universidade do Porto, Portugal

RESEARCH SUMMARY

Among seafood species, cephalopods represent one of the ecologically and commercially most interesting classes. They are active predators and simultaneously important prey items for mammals. Cephalopods are part of the traditional diet of Japan, Korea, Argentina, Taiwan and China, and of coastal communities of southern Europe, such as Spain, Portugal, Morocco, Mauritania, Greece and Italy. Their importance to fisheries is expected to increase with the decline in traditional finfish stocks across the globe.

The cephalopods capacity to accumulate contaminants and to grow and reproduce in polluted milieus is well described in the literature. Among these contaminants, polycyclic aromatic hydrocarbons (PAHs) deserve special attention due to the potential cytotoxicity, mutagenicity, and carcinogenicity presented by some compounds. Additionally, in aquatic food chains, cephalopods have the poorest metabolic capacity to metabolize PAHs. Although the highest concentrations of PAHs may be found in digestive glands of cephalopods, edible parts, i.e., arms and mantle, are the most commonly eaten by humans and the total amount of toxic elements in these tissues may still be significant. With the aim of minimizing harmful effects on human health, the European Union established a maximum level of 5.0 μg/kg wet weight for benzo(a)pyrene (the marker used for PAHs carcinogenic risks) in cephalopods other than smoked (Commission Regulation (EC) 1881/2006). This chapter will present the main characteristics of cephalopods, the major PAH sources of the marine environment and

---

* REQUIMTE, Instituto Superior de Engenharia do Porto, R. Dr. António Bernardino de Almeida 431, 4200-072 Porto, Portugal; sbm@isep.ipp.pt
# REQUIMTE, Dep. Ciências Químicas, Faculdade de Farmácia, Universidade do Porto, Rua Jorge Viterbo Ferreira 228, 4050-313 Porto, Portugal; beatoliv@ff.up.pt

review the reported levels of PAHs in cephalopod species, in order to assess their status of contamination and the associated public health risks through their consumption.

In: Chemistry Research Summaries Volume 12
Editor: Lucille Monaco Cacioppo

ISBN: 978-1-61668-757-1
© 2014 Nova Science Publishers, Inc.

Chapter 82

CHILDREN ENVIRONMENTALLY EXPOSED TO POLYCYCLIC AROMATIC HYDROCARBONS ARE AT RISK OF GENOTOXIC EFFECTS

M. Sánchez-Guerra and B. Quintanilla-Vega[*]
Departamento de Toxicología, CINVESTAV-IPN, México, D. F., México

RESEARCH SUMMARY

Polycyclic aromatic hydrocarbons (PAHs) are generated during pyrolysis of organic material. Exposure to these ubiquitous environmental contaminants is a public health problem in cities with high industrial activity and vehicular traffic as well as in rural areas due to biomass combustion. An estimate of 90% of rural populations in developing countries uses biomass as energy source, where PAH exposure can be extremely high by means of their main exposure biomarker, 1-hydroxipyrene (1-OHP) in urine. Critical scenarios in children have shown PAH levels as high as 17 μmol 1-OHP/mol creatinine. Another disturbing PAH source for children is indoor exposure to smoke from smoking parents. PAHs are human carcinogen compounds and infant populations are most vulnerable to their toxicity, highlighting the risk at which they are exposed. The genotoxic properties of PAHs are mediated by their metabolism generating reactive metabolites that interact with DNA. Several biomarkers of DNA damage such as increased frequencies of chromosomal aberrations and micronucleus, and hemoglobin and DNA adducts have been reported in children and newborns exposed to airborne pollutants. Furthermore, epidemiological studies have found increased risk of leukemia and nervous system tumors in children with high exposure to environmental pollution and research has suggested that cancer susceptibility is higher if the exposure to carcinogenic compounds occurs during fetal and childhood periods. To date, there are no PAH exposure limits to protect general population´s health, and unfortunately, in

[*] Correspondence should be addressed to: Betzabet Quintanilla-Vega Address: Ave. IPN 2508, Col. Zacatenco, Mexico City, 07360, Mexico Phone: (52)+55-57473800 Ext. 5446 Fax (52)+55-57473395 E-mail: mquintan@cinvestav.mx

most developing countries there are no strict regulations to control environmental pollutants that additionally put at risk children´s health.

In: Chemistry Research Summaries Volume 12
Editor: Lucille Monaco Cacioppo

ISBN: 978-1-61668-757-1
© 2014 Nova Science Publishers, Inc.

Chapter 83

HYDROXYLATED NITRO POLYCYCLIC AROMATIC COMPOUNDS: ATMOSPHERIC OCCURRENCE AND HEALTH IMPACTS

Takayuki Kameda[*], *Ayuko Akiyama, Akira Toriba,*
Ning Tang and Kazuichi Hayakawa
Institute of Medical, Pharmaceutical and Health Sciences, Kanazawa University,
Kakuma-machi, Kanazawa, Ishikawa, Japan

RESEARCH SUMMARY

Polycyclic aromatic compounds, which are ubiquitous atmospheric pollutants with toxic properties, are produced from chemical reactions of their parent compounds in the atmosphere as well as from a wide variety of anthropogenic sources such as fuel combustions. The present report is mainly concerned with atmospheric occurrence and health effects of hydroxylated nitro polycyclic aromatic compounds such as hydroxynitropyrenes (OHNPs) and hydroxynitrofluoranthenes (OHNFs). The formation of OHNPs and OHNFs *via* photochemical reactions of their parent nitro polycyclic aromatic hydrocarbons (NPAHs) was demonstrated using a UV irradiation system. The photoreaction of 1-nitropyrene (1-NP) gave products that were hydroxy-substituted at position 1 and mononitro-substituted at positions 2, 3, 5, 6 and 8 (1-hydroxy-x-nitropyrenes (1-OH-x-NPs); x = 2, 3, 5, 6, and 8). 1-OH-2-NP and 1-OH-5-NP were identified in ambient airborne particles. On the contrary, these two OHNP isomers have not been found in samples of diesel exhaust particles (DEP). The concentrations of the other OHNP isomers in the DEP samples were much lower than the concentration of 1-NP, which is a representative NPAH that is emitted directly from combustion sources. On the other hand, significantly higher concentration ratios of ΣOHNP (= 1-OH-3-NP + 1-OH-6-NP + 1-OH-8-NP) to 1-NP were observed in ambient airborne particles than in the DEP samples. The photoreaction of 2-nitrofluoranthene (2-NF) also gave a product that was hydroxynitro-

[*] Corresponding author: Takayuki Kameda, Institute of Medical, Pharmaceutical and Health Sciences, Kanazawa University, Kakuma-machi, Kanazawa, Ishikawa 920-1192, Japan, Phone: +81-76-234-4458, Fax: +81-76-234-4456, email: kameda@p.kanazawa-u.ac.jp

substituted. Moreover, we detected an OHNF isomer, which was found in the 2-NF photoreaction products, in soluble organic fractions of ambient airborne particles. The atmospheric concentration of the OHNF isomer was estimated to be comparable to that of 1-OH-3-NP, but lower than that of 1-OH-6-NP by a factor of 10. These results support the idea that atmospheric OHNPs and OHNFs are predominantly formed *via* secondary formation processes, i.e., photochemical reactions of their parent NPAHs are expected to have a significant effect on the occurrence of OHNPs and OHNFs in the atmosphere. Endocrine disrupting activities of the five isomers of OHNP were evaluated by yeast two-hybrid assay. OHNPs did not exhibit androgenic activity but exhibited estrogenic, antiestrogenic, and antiandrogenic activities. 1-OH-6-NP showed the strongest estrogenic activity among the five OHNP isomers examined in this study. On the contrary, 1-OH-5-NP exhibited the strongest antiestrogenic and antiandrogenic activities of the five isomers. These findings point out the necessity for detailed investigation of environmental distributions of hydroxylated nitro polycyclic aromatic compounds as well as the parent NPAHs.

In: Chemistry Research Summaries Volume 12   ISBN: 978-1-61668-757-1
Editor: Lucille Monaco Cacioppo   © 2014 Nova Science Publishers, Inc.

Chapter 84

ANALYSIS OF PAHS IN ENVIRONMENTAL SOLID SAMPLES

Nobuyasu Itoh
National Metrology Institute of Japan (NMIJ), National Institute
of Advanced Industrial Science and Technology (AIST), Japan

RESEARCH SUMMARY

Polycyclic aromatic hydrocarbons (PAHs) are widely distributed throughout the world; thus, it is essential to collect and accumulate analytical results from many groups and researchers. The comparability of PAH analytical results from different researchers is important for reliable evaluation of the environmental distributions and fate of PAHs. However, the reliability of the results is sometimes ignored, and biased results may lead to misunderstanding of the fates of PAHs in the environment. Here, I will review analyses of PAHs, from sample pretreatment to instrumental measurement, and provide useful information for obtaining reliable analytical results.

The sampling framework is the first step to obtaining reliable results. Sample pretreatment and extraction of PAHs from environmental samples are essential and important processes because reliable PAH concentrations cannot be obtained if this step is insufficient. A subsequent clean-up step is also important, but in some cases this step can be ignored for clean extracts. Measurement of PAHs using analytical instruments is the final step of the analytical procedure, and it is also an important step because PAHs vary widely in their physical/chemical properties and the separation of some structural isomers is difficult under conventional conditions. I will also provide information regarding the certified reference materials that are suitable for the validation of analytical results.

In: Chemistry Research Summaries Volume 12
Editor: Lucille Monaco Cacioppo

ISBN: 978-1-61668-757-1
© 2014 Nova Science Publishers, Inc.

Chapter 85

EXPOSURE TO POLYCYCLIC AROMATIC HYDROCARBONS AND THE ASSOCIATED HEALTH RISKS IN SCHOOLCHILDREN: A REVIEW

Marta Oliveira[1,2], Klara Slezakova[1,2], C. Delerue-Matos[2], Maria do Carmo Pereira[1] and Simone Morais[2]*

[1]LEPAE, Departamento de Engenharia Química, Faculdade de Engenharia, Universidade do Porto, Porto, Portugal
[2]REQUIMTE, Instituto Superior de Engenharia do Porto, Porto, Portugal

RESEARCH SUMMARY

Up to this date, numerous studies have associated exposure to PAHs with various health problems. The increasing awareness of the health hazards posed by PAHs present in indoor air has led to many preventive and restorative indoor air quality programs being implemented worldwide. Typically, the health concerns of PAHs are focused on their potential cytotoxicity, mutagenicity, and carcinogenicity in humans. Whereas the health risks of adult exposure cannot be neglected, children are much more susceptible as some studies showed that poor indoor air causes adverse health effects in children regardless of their health status. As children spend much of their time at schools, these environments may represent the major contributor to children's exposure to air pollutants; conditions found in schools may strongly impact on the respective health outcomes. So far there are only few data on indoor PAHs exposure and the respective health risks. Additionally, studies on levels and health risks associated with exposure to PAHs in schoolchildren are scarce. Protection against detrimental action of air pollutants requires reliable information about their levels of exposure. Thus this chapter is dedicated to schoolchildren exposure to PAHs and the associated health risks. A brief discussion on characteristics of PAHs is given, covering their sources as well as their health impacts. Available information on levels of exposure in schools is then summarized and the main results from existent epidemiological studies on children reported.

* Email: sbm@isep.ipp.pt

In: Chemistry Research Summaries Volume 12   ISBN: 978-1-61668-757-1
Editor: Lucille Monaco Cacioppo   © 2014 Nova Science Publishers, Inc.

Chapter 86

CHEMICAL AND ELECTRONIC PROPERTIES OF POLYCYCLIC AROMATIC HYDROCARBONS: A REVIEW

Sergio Manzetti[*]
FJORDFORSK Environmental and Health Sciences,
Flåm, Norway

RESEARCH SUMMARY

Polycyclic aromatic hydrocarbons are ubiquitous environmental pollutants with peculiar chemical characters, which can be generalized as aromatic and is represented by the geometrical foundation for all PAHs: the benzene ring. However considerable differences from monocyclic to polycyclic states occur and medium-sized and larger PAHs can differ chemically from the small aromatic compounds, benzene, naphthalene and anthracene. This review investigates and reports on the molecular properties, differences, and degrees of aromaticity and reactivity of PAHs, in addition to their electronic properties and resonance states. This chapter serves to supply knowledge on PAHs for chemical and environmental chemistry purposes.

[*] www.fjordforsk.no

In: Chemistry Research Summaries Volume 12
Editor: Lucille Monaco Cacioppo

ISBN: 978-1-61668-757-1
© 2014 Nova Science Publishers, Inc.

Chapter 87

MUTAGENIC POTENTIAL AND PROFILE OF PAHS IN SOILS CONTAMINATED BY WOOD PRESERVATIVES: EFFECTS ON THE ENVIRONMENT AND ON HUMAN HEALTH

Vera Maria Ferrão Vargas[1,2]*, Roberta de Souza Pohren[1,2], Flávio da Silva Júnior Souza[1], Jorge Willian Moreira[1], Jocelita Vaz Rocha[1], Cristiani Rigotti Vaz[1], Daniel Derrossi Meyer[1] and Karen Leal[1]

[1]Programa de Pesquisas Ambientais, Fundação Estadual de Proteção Ambiental Henrique Luís Roessler (FEPAM), Porto Alegre, RS, Brazil
[2]Programa de Pós-graduação em Ecologia, Universidade Federal do Rio Grande do Sul (UFRGS), Porto Alegre, RS, Brazil

RESEARCH SUMMARY

Many agricultural and industrial practices have contributed to modifying all environmental compartments.

This includes the soil, often considered a deposit for wastes, which has received tons of contaminants directly and indirectly, altering its composition, and turning it inappropriately into a pollutant reservoir. It may thus become a potential source of contamination for the other compartments. Different chemicals were used in the area of study, an inactivated old wood preservation plant, including a pentachlorophenol solution in oil and/or creosote oil. Creosote is oil composed approximately 85% of polycyclic aromatic hydrocarbons (PAHs), whose toxicity persists in the environment, presenting possible carcinogenicity. However, it is acknowledged that other pollutants of the aromatic polycyclic class contribute significantly to toxicity in the contaminated environments, such as the nitrated PAHs (Nitro-PAHs). These present highly toxic chemical characteristics and may qualify potential risks existing in the

---

* Email: ecorisco@fepam.rs.gov.br

area. Until recently, most classical studies on the evaluation and control of environmental quality were exclusively based on physical and chemical parameters. This approach, although essential, does not sufficiently characterize environmental contamination, since it does not take into account the possible interaction between contaminants, environmental matrix and biota. It is thus essential to perform a broader evaluation of the impact of these multiple stressors. Bioassays are an important tool, supplying additional information about human ecological risks and allowing the integration of effects of bioavailable concentrations. Among these assays are those that evaluate the potential risk of these complex mixtures for genotoxicity, such as Salmonella/microsome or the Ames Test. Therefore, the study attempted to define the contamination of soil samples from the industrial area of the contaminated site, focusing on the PAHs profile of the samples and their relationship with the mutagenic responses obtained. Based on the soil samples, fractionated organic extracts of the PAHs and nitro-PAHs were prepared. In order to evaluate mutagenesis, specific strains were tested that measure molecular damage by frameshift error (TA98, TA97a) and base pair substitution (TA100), in the presence and absence of liver metabolization of rats (S9mix) besides the YGs 1041 and 1042, specific for nitrocompounds. The results indicated the presence of different PAHs, as well as their biological effects through biomarkers in the samples analyzed. This approach, evaluating different fractions of the complex environmental matrix, allowed to define the more aggressive classes of compounds, indicating the presence of potential effects of these contaminants. It is a promising alternative, among the soil quality indicators, to be used for evaluations of ecological and human risk.

Supported by CNPq 555187/2008-0;576027/2008-2.

In: Chemistry Research Summaries Volume 12   ISBN: 978-1-61668-757-1
Editor: Lucille Monaco Cacioppo   © 2014 Nova Science Publishers, Inc.

Chapter 88

PHASE BEHAVIOR AND THERMOCHEMICAL PROPERTIES OF POLYCYCLIC AROMATIC HYDROCARBONS AND THEIR DERIVATIVES

Jinxia Fu[*1], James W. Rice[2] and Eric M. Suuberg[2]*
[1] Brown University Department of Chemistry, Providence, Rhode Island, US
[2] Brown University School of Engineering, Providence, Rhode Island, US

RESEARCH SUMMARY

Polycyclic aromatic hydrocarbons are compounds resulting from incomplete combustion and many fuel processing operations, and they are commonly found as subsurface environmental contaminants at sites of former manufactured gas plants. 16 PAHs are classified as priority pollutants by the US EPA. Recently, interest has also increased in PAH derivatives, such as halogenated PAHs (HPAHs) and heteroatomic PAHs, due to their biological activity and health effects. Just as for PAHs, the HPAHs have been reported to occur in various matrices, such as urban air, snow, tap water, kraft pulp mill waste, fly and bottom ash from waste incinerators, and electronic waste. The knowledge of their phase behavior and thermochemical properties is key to predicting their fate and transport in the environment.

In this chapter, a compendium of the vapor pressure, and temperatures and enthalpies of phase change of the 16 priority PAHs and the HPAHs with one or two halogen substitutions is presented. Phase change enthalpies, including for fusion and sublimation, are summarized. Enthalpies and entropies of sublimation of these compounds were determined via application of the Clausius–Clapeyron equation. For most PAHs, sufficient data are available to permit the evaluation of the reliability of the measurements. The measured vapor pressure values were extrapolated to 298.15 K. The HPAH data were also compared with PAH values to study the influence of halogen substitution on vapor pressures and enthalpies of phase change.

---

[*] corresponding author

In: Chemistry Research Summaries Volume 12   ISBN: 978-1-61668-757-1
Editor: Lucille Monaco Cacioppo   © 2014 Nova Science Publishers, Inc.

Chapter 89

PAH-DNA Adducts in Non-Smoking Inhabitants of Mexico City

W. A. García-Suástegui[1], A. Huerta-Chagoya[1], M. M. Pratt[2], K. John[b], P. Petrosyan[1], J. Rubio[1], M. C. Poirier[2] and M. E. Gonsebatt[*,1]

[1]Department of Genetic Medicine and Environmental Toxicology,
Instituto de Investigaciones Biomédicas, Universidad Nacional Autónoma de México,
Mexico City, México
[2]Carcinogen-DNA Interactions Section, National Cancer Institute,
National Institutes of Health, Bethesda, Maryland, US

RESEARCH SUMMARY

The Mexico City metropolitan area (MCMA) is one of the most densely populated cities in the world, with nearly 20 million inhabitants. One consequence of this urban concentration is the daily circulation of more than 4 million vehicles that generate elevated levels of polycyclic aromatic hydrocarbons (PAHs), which are not monitored or regulated. Several studies indicate that PAH levels in the MCMA ambient air are above those reported in other highly polluted cities, particularly during the winter season as a result of thermal inversions and the lack of rain. Exposure to PAHs can be ascertained by the determination of adducts on the DNA, which are lesions considered to be associated with an enhanced risk of cancer formation. Using a chemiluminescence immunoassay with an antiserum elicited against DNA modified with benzo[a]pyrene (B[a]P), we performed a monitoring study to determine the levels of PAH-DNA adducts during winter and the subsequent summer. The assay was performed on DNA isolated from peripheral blood lymphocytes from young non-smoking inhabitants of the MCMA. The levels of PAH-DNA adducts were higher in winter than in other times of the year, and were associated with airborne levels of particulate matter in the

---

* Corresponding author: M. E. Gonsebatt, Department of Genetic Medicine and Environmental Toxicology, Instituto de Investigaciones Biomédicas, Universidad Nacional Autónoma de México, A.P. 70-228, Ciudad Universitaria 04510, Mexico City, México.

most highly affected areas. Our observations indicate the need for air quality standards and regulations for PAHs in the MCMA, as well as improvement of the strategies to reduce vehicle emissions.

In: Chemistry Research Summaries Volume 12   ISBN: 978-1-61668-757-1
Editor: Lucille Monaco Cacioppo   © 2014 Nova Science Publishers, Inc.

Chapter 90

DETERMINATION OF POLYCYCLIC AROMATIC HYDROCARBONS IN DRINKING WATER SOURCES

Sandra Sanches[1,2], Joana Ricardo[1], Maria C. Leitão[2],
*Maria T. Barreto Crespo[1,2] and Vanessa J. Pereira[*1,2]*
[1]Instituto de Biologia Experimental e Tecnológica, Oeiras, Portugal
[2]Instituto de Tecnologia Química e Biológica, Universidade Nova de Lisboa,
Oeiras, Portugal

RESEARCH SUMMARY

Ultra-high-speed liquid chromatography was compared with traditional high performance liquid chromatography for the analysis of polycyclic aromatic hydrocarbons (PAHs) considered as priority pollutants by the European Water Framework Directive. Ultra-high-speed liquid chromatography significantly increased the speed of analysis while considerably decreasing the solvent consumption and waste generation. Different solid phase extraction cartridges and procedures were evaluated using matrices with very different compositions. The percent recoveries obtained after spiking different matrices with the selected PAHs show that the tested procedures enable their detection at ng/L levels in real water matrices and that the use of an organic modifier clearly enhances the solid phase extraction efficiency.

* Corresponding author: Vanessa J. Pereira, Instituto de Biologia Experimental e Tecnológica, Instituto de Tecnologia Química e Biológica/Universidade Nova de Lisboa, Av. da República (EAN), 2781-901 Oeiras, Portugal, E-mail address: vanessap@itqb.unl.pt, Phone number: + 351214469568, Fax number: + 351 21 4421161

In: Chemistry Research Summaries Volume 12
Editor: Lucille Monaco Cacioppo

ISBN: 978-1-61668-757-1
© 2014 Nova Science Publishers, Inc.

Chapter 91

ALKALI HALIDE CLUSTERS: EXPERIMENT AND THEORY

Francisco Fernandez-Lima,[1] Enio F. da Silveira[2] and Marco Antonio Chaer Nascimento[3]*

[1]Department of Chemistry and Biochemistry,
Florida International University, Miami, Florida, US
[2]Department of Physics, Pontifícia Universidade Católica,
Rio de Janeiro, Brazil
[3]Chemistry Institute, Universidade Federal do Rio de Janeiro,
Rio de Janeiro, Brazil

RESEARCH SUMMARY

The study of alkali halide cluster and cluster-assembled materials has revealed that they present unique physical and chemical properties that are quite different from those of the corresponding bulk crystals. In particular, alkali (X) halide (Y) cluster ions are commonly observed in the forms $(XY)_n^{-1,0,+1}$, $(XY)_n X^{0,+1}$ and $(XY)_n Y^{0,-1}$ and their properties vary as a function of their size, charge and nature of atomic constituents, i.e., their properties are intimately related to the X and Y constituent electronic densities. A detailed characterization of each member of a cluster ion series permits a better understanding of the cluster properties. Theoretical calculations can be very useful in predicting atomic and molecular properties or parameters which might be difficult to verify experimentally such as binding energies, ionization potentials, vibration frequencies, and fragmentation patterns of atomic and molecular clusters. They can also be helpful in the interpretation of experiments by providing details of the geometrical configurations and of the electronic density distribution. In the present chapter, we will mainly focus on experimental data of charged species emitted from alkali halide targets and theoretical predictions of their relative stability, fragmentation

---

* Corresponding author: Francisco Fernandez-Lima, Assist. Prof. Florida International University, Department of Chemistry and Biochemistry, CP-312 11200 SW 8th Str. Miami, Florida 33199; Ph: 305-348-2037; Fax: 305-348-3772; E-mail: fernandf@fiu.edu.

energies and charge distributions. We will cover small cluster systems (e.g., $n = 1 - 5$) to nanometric size clusters (e.g., $n = 20 - 40$).

In: Chemistry Research Summaries Volume 12
Editor: Lucille Monaco Cacioppo

ISBN: 978-1-61668-757-1
© 2014 Nova Science Publishers, Inc.

Chapter 92

Synthesis, Characterization and Influence of Electrolyte Solutions towards the Electrical Properties of Nylon-6,6 Nickel Carbonate Membrane: Test for the Theory of Uni-ionic Potential Based on Thermodynamics of Irreversible Processes

Tanvir Arfin[1], and Faruq Mohammad[2,3]*

[1]PGM Group, Chemical Resource Beneficiation (CRB) Research
Focus Area, North-West University, South Africa
[2]Department of Environmental Toxicology,
Southern University and A&M College, Baton Rouge, Louisiana, US
[3]Center for Advanced Microstructures and Devices,
Louisiana State University, Baton Rouge, Louisiana, US

Research Summary

In this study, the nano-crystalline organic-inorganic composite nylon-6,6 nickel carbonate membrane was synthesised, subsequent to which (a) the physico-chemical characteristics of the membrane was evaluated by employing ATR-FTIR, SEM, EDX, TEM,TGA, XRD, and porosity measurements, and (b) membrane potential measurements were carried out using different concentrations of KCl, NaCl and LiCl 1:1 electrolyte solutions($2.5 \times 10^{-2} \leq c$ (M)$\leq 1 \times 10^{0}$).For the potential measurements, the high C_2 concentrations of the electrolyte were maintained on one side of the membrane and low C_1

---

*Corresponding Author. Tel.: +27 (0) 18 299 1576; Fax: +27 (0) 18 299 1667.Email address: tanvirarfin@ymail.com (T. Arfin), faruq_mohammad@subr.edu (F. Mohammad).

concentration of the same electrolyte on the other side of the membrane, where the solution-concentration ratio (C_2/C_1) was maintained at 10 and the membrane potentials found to be higher at low pH values. Also, we observed the positive membrane potentials for the composite membrane and is an indication of the membrane to be negatively charged and this potential found to be dependent of cation selectivity and is decreasing in the order LiCl>NaCl>KCl. At low electrolyte concentrations, the membrane potential found to be high and with increase of concentration, the membrane potential deceased. In addition to the potential measurements, the successful application of Teorell-Meyer and Sievers (TMS), Kobatake et al. and Nagasawa et al. theories were also employed to estimate the charge density of the membrane immersed in different electrolytes and it was found that the charge densities decreased in the order KCl>NaCl>LiCl for 1:1 electrolytes. The extended TMS theory was used to investigate the transference numbers, mobility ratio, distribution coefficients, charge effectiveness, perm selectivity and concentration of fixed charge for 1:1 electrolyte solutions.

In: Chemistry Research Summaries Volume 12
Editor: Lucille Monaco Cacioppo

ISBN: 978-1-61668-757-1
© 2014 Nova Science Publishers, Inc.

Chapter 93

NUCLEOPHILIC SUBSTITUTION AND PALLADIUM-CATALYZED COUPLING MECHANISMS OF AROMATIC HALIDES

Linjun Shao, Kai Chen, Minfeng Zeng, Chen Wang, Chenze Qi and Xian-Man Zhang[*]
Department of Chemistry, University of Shaoxing, Shaoxing, Zhejiang Province, People's Republic of China

RESEARCH SUMMARY

Unactivated aromatic halides typically do not react with nucleophiles unless submitted to extremely drastic reaction conditions. The extremely low reactivities of aromatic halides can be attributed to their sTable aromatic π electron structure. But the unactivated aromatic halides can readily undergo radical nucleophilic substitution ($S_{RN}1$) and palladium-catalyzed reactions under relatively mild conditions. The remarkable enhancement of the aromatic halide reactivities has been attributed to their activation by electron transfer and/or palladium oxidative insertion. The palladium-catalyzed coupling of aromatic halides has been become as one of the most important chemical transformations for the construction of carbon-carbon chemical bonds in synthetic organic chemistry. The related reaction mechanisms and their synthetic applications will be discussed with an emphasis on the author's research interests.

---

[*] E-mail: xian-man.zhang@usx.edu.cn and xianmanzhang@yahoo.com.

In: Chemistry Research Summaries Volume 12
Editor: Lucille Monaco Cacioppo

ISBN: 978-1-61668-757-1
© 2014 Nova Science Publishers, Inc.

Chapter 94

DISLOCATION PINNED BY A MONOVALENT ION IN VARIOUS ALKALI HALIDE CRYSTALS

Y. Kohzuki[*]

Oshima National College of Maritime Technology,
Oshima-gun, Yamaguchi, Japan

RESEARCH SUMMARY

Part I. Various Models between a Dislocation and the Monovalent Cation

The force-distance ($F(x)$) relation, which represents the model overcoming a weak obstacle by a dislocation with the help of thermal fluctuations, is described here for short-range obstacle less than about 10 atomic diameters. Furthermore, the three models (the square, the parabolic, and the triangular $F(x)$) taking account of the Friedel relation are investigated with respect to the relation between effective stress and temperature for $KCl:Li^+$ and $KCl:Na^+$ single crystals. On the three force-distance relations, the value of T_c is almost the same irrespective of the kind of force-distance relation for both the specimens, and the value of T_c (254~257 K) for $KCl:Li^+$ is obviously small in comparison with that (266~271 K) for $KCl:Na^+$. T_c is the critical temperature at which the effective stress becomes zero and a dislocation breaks away from the defects of cubic symmetry around Li^+ or Na^+ only with the help of thermal activation.

Part II. Characteristics on the Breakaway of a Dislocation from the Monovalent Cation

The energy for the breakaway of a dislocation from the monovalent cation is obtained through the slope of linear relationship of reciprocal of temperature ($1/T$) versus

---
[*] Corresponding author's email: kouzuki@oshima-k.ac.jp

$\tau_{p1}(\Delta\ln\dot{\varepsilon}/\Delta\tau')_p$. Here τ_{p1} represents the effective stress and $(\Delta\ln\dot{\varepsilon}/\Delta\tau')_p$ the reciprocal of strain-rate sensitivity due to the additive cations when a dislocation moves forward with the help of oscillation during plastic deformation. Analyzing this result, it would be deduced that the breaking angle ϕ_0 is around 178° and $(L/L_0) \approx 7.0$ for KCl: Li$^+$ or Na$^+$ single crystals. L is the average length of dislocation segments and L_0 the average spacing of monovalent cations on a slip plane.

Part III. Breaking Angle of an Anion as Obstacle for Moving Dislocation

The breaking angle ϕ_0, at which a dislocation breaks away from a weak obstacle at the temperature of 0 K, measures the strength of the obstacle-dislocation interaction. The ϕ_0 ranges 173° to 177° for the various alkali halides single crystals (NaCl:Br$^-$, NaBr: Cl$^-$ or I$^-$, KCl: Br$^-$ or I$^-$, and RbCl: Br$^-$ or I$^-$). The values of (L/L_0) were found to be within 4.05 to 5.87 there. L is the average length of dislocation segments and L_0 the average spacing of monovalent anions on a slip plane.

In: Chemistry Research Summaries Volume 12   ISBN: 978-1-61668-757-1
Editor: Lucille Monaco Cacioppo   © 2014 Nova Science Publishers, Inc.

Chapter 95

THE NONLINEAR ELASTIC PROPERTIES AND GRÜNEISEN CONSTANTS OF ALKALI HALIDE[*]

X. Z. Wu[†], L. L. Liu, R. Wang, C. B. Li, S. H. Wu and H. F. Feng

College of Physics and Institute for Structure and Function,
Chongqing University, Chongqing, P. R. China

RESEARCH SUMMARY

The second-order elastic constants (SOECs) and third-order elastic constants (TOECs) of the alkali halides (LiF, NaF, KF, LiCl, NaCl and KCl) with NaCl structure is presented using the density functional theory (DFT) and homogeneous deformation method. The k-points and the cutoff energy are given reliable verification while TOECs are concerned. From the nonlinear least-square fitting, the elastic constants are extracted from a polynomial fit to the calculated strain-energy data. Both the SOECs and TOECs are in agreement with the available experimental and previous results. The Lagrangian stress is changing linearly for small Lagrangian strain and it is found that the nonlinear effects play an important role while the finite strains are larger than approximately 0.025. The pressure derivatives of SOECs are calculated directly using the TOECs, which is used to discuss roughly the phase transition pressure of alkali halide. The Grüneisen constants of long-wavelength acoustic modes characterizing the anharmonic properties of alkali halide are also presented.

[*] Project Supported by the Natural Science Foundation of China (11104361).
[†] E-mail address: xiaozhiwu@cqu.edu.cn

In: Chemistry Research Summaries Volume 12
Editor: Lucille Monaco Cacioppo

ISBN: 978-1-61668-757-1
© 2014 Nova Science Publishers, Inc.

Chapter 96

METALS IN LIQUID HELIUM: DISCONTINUOUS YIELDING, STRESS DROPS, AND STRENGTH

E. V. Vorob'ev, V. A. Strizhalo and T. V. Anpilogova

G. S. Pisarenko Institute for Problems of Strength,
National Academy of Sciences of Ukraine, Ukraine

RESEARCH SUMMARY

The mechanical behavior of metals under load in liquid helium is studied. The mechanisms and manifestations of low-temperature discontinuous yielding (jerky flow) are considered. The accompanying thermal effects are evaluated by analyzing energy conversion and deformation behavior. Criteria for new limiting states that occur during discontinuous yielding are established.

A two-parameter (temperature and stress) criterion of instability of plastic deformation of metals is formulated. It can be used to calculate the maximum critical temperature and the critical stress at given temperature. The influence of the loading conditions and design/technology factors on the discontinuous yielding characteristics and mechanical properties of some steels and alloys at a temperature of 4 K was studied experimentally. Prestrain, as well as stress concentrators in combination with low rigidity of the structure or supercritical strain rates may cause fracture of a structural member. A method for the experimental simulation of a strain jump at room temperature is developed and shown to be capable of reproducing and studying effects similar to those observed in liquid helium. A nonlinear multiparameter mathematical model of a strain jump is set up.

The dependence of strain jumps on the mechanical characteristics of the material, the dynamic characteristics of the testing machine, rated strain rate, and scale effect is established numerically for the widest possible ranges of these factors. A method for determining ultimate stresses with allowance for the low-temperature hardening of metals and the effects of discontinuous yielding is proposed. Recommendations on how to improve the tensile test method for metals at temperatures below 20 K are formulated.

In: Chemistry Research Summaries Volume 12
Editor: Lucille Monaco Cacioppo

Chapter 97

THE USE OF HELIUM WITH OXYGEN AT PRESSURE AS A BREATHING GAS MIXTURE

*Jean-Claude Rostain**
Aix-Marseille University, UMR-MD2,
Faculté de Médecine Nord, Marseille, France

RESEARCH SUMMARY

The use of compressed air or nitrogen-oxygen mixture in diving induce from 30 metres of sea water several neurological and psychomotor disturbances due to the increase of partial pressure of nitrogen and to its narcotic potency called nitrogen narcosis. To avoid these disturbances, nitrogen has been replaced by helium, an inert gas with a low narcotic potency in relationship with its very low lipid solubility. With helium-oxygen synthetic gas mixture, depths higher than 50 metres or pressure higher of 0.5 MPa have been reached up to 6.1MPa. However, from 1 MPa physiological and neurophysiological changes different from the symptoms of nitrogen narcosis have been reported. In man, these changes consist of electroencephalographic modifications from 1MPa, occurrence of tremor and sleep disturbances from around 2MPa, myoclonia and dysmetria from 4MPa, and in experimental animals, epileptic seizures for pressure higher than 8MPa. Theses disturbances have been regrouped in a high pressure nervous syndrome (HPNS), as helium did not seem implicated in these disruptions. Indeed, if helium has narcotic properties, the signs and symptoms will be similar to or worse than 0.9MPa compressed air at about 4.1MPa. However owing to antagonism of the weak narcotic effect of helium by the increased pressure (called the pressure reversal effect) there is no helium narcosis. However, in the light of results obtained with narcotic gases added to helium oxygen mixture, such as nitrogen or hydrogen, mood changes and some somesthetic hallucinations reported at pressure higher than 4-5 MPa could be in relationship with a narcotic effect of helium rather than a pressure effect. Moreover hallucinatory behaviours have been reported in monkeys in helium oxygen mixture for pressure of 8MPa and above.

* Tel. 33 4 9169 89 06; Fax. 33 4 91 65 38 51; jean-claude.rostain@univ-amu.fr.

Neuropharmacological and neurochemical studies (microdialysis and voltammetry) performed with helium-oxygen mixture at pressure have demonstrated changes in amino-acid (gama-amino-butyric acid and glutamate) and monoamine (dopamine and serotonin) neurotransmission regulations at the level of basal ganglia, brain structures implicated in the regulation of the motor, loco-motor and cognitive processes.

In: Chemistry Research Summaries Volume 12
Editor: Lucille Monaco Cacioppo

ISBN: 978-1-61668-757-1
© 2014 Nova Science Publishers, Inc.

Chapter 98

PHYSICS AND CHEMISTRY OF HELIUM CLUSTERS AND DROPLETS

J. Peter Toennies[*]

Max-Planck-Institut für Dynamik und Selbstorganisation,
Göttingen, Germany

RESEARCH SUMMARY

Many microscopic properties of the only natural superfluid element helium have only become available within the last 18 years through a number of novel experiments. The diffraction of matter-waves of small helium clusters have established the unusually large bond distance (5.2 nm) and extremely weak binding energy (10^{-7} eV) of the dimer and other exotic properties of small helium clusters. The high resolution spectroscopy of closed shell chromophore molecules attached to small clusters or embedded inside large superfluid droplets have revealed that as a result of superfluidity molecules rotate virtually without friction and that only a hand-full of He atoms are required. These and a number of other experiments demonstrate that helium droplets are the most gentle and coldest of all cryomatrices with enormous potential for a wide range of future applications.

---

[*] Email: jtoenni@gwdg.de.

In: Chemistry Research Summaries Volume 12
Editor: Lucille Monaco Cacioppo

ISBN: 978-1-61668-757-1
© 2014 Nova Science Publishers, Inc.

Chapter 99

INTERACTION OF HELIUM ATOMS AND IONS WITH MATTER

Ya. A. Teplova[*], N. V. Novikov and Yu. A. Belkova

Scobeltsyn Institute of Nuclear Physics,
Lomonosov Moscow State University, Moscow, Russia

RESEARCH SUMMARY

The electron loss and electron capture cross sections, equilibrium target thickness, energy loss and ranges are studied experimentally for helium atoms and helium ions with velocities $(2.6 - 20) \times 10^8$ cm/s in various targets. The energy, angular and charge distributions of helium ions and atoms reflected from a metal surface at grazing incidence are measured at the energy 250 and 300 keV. On the bases of experimental data some effects of ion interaction with matter are discussed theoretically (nonmonotonic dependence of range, energy loss, and charge-changing cross sections on nuclear charges of the colliding particles, density effects in gaseous and solid targets etc.). The experimental values are given by figures and by tables in appendix.

---

[*] Corresponding author. e-mail: teplova@anna19.sinp.msu.ru.

In: Chemistry Research Summaries Volume 12   ISBN: 978-1-61668-757-1
Editor: Lucille Monaco Cacioppo   © 2014 Nova Science Publishers, Inc.

Chapter 100

POSTSEISMIC LEAKAGE OF MANTLE AND CRUSTAL HELIUM FROM SEISMICALLY ACTIVE REGIONS

Koji Umeda, Koichi Asamori, Ryo Komatsu,*
Chifumi Kakuta, Sunao Kanazawa,
Atusi Ninomiya, Tomohiro Kusano and Kazuo Kobori
Tono Geoscientific Research Unit,
Geological Isolation Research and Development Directorate,
Japan Atomic Energy Agency, Jorinji, Izumi, Toki, Japan

RESEARCH SUMMARY

It is well known that mantle degassing does not occur homogeneously over the Earth's surface. The elevated $^3He/^4He$ ratios found in volcanic regions and tectonically active areas are higher than the atmospheric values. The anomalous helium isotopic ratios have been interpreted to transfer mantle volatiles into the crust by processes or mechanisms such as magmatic intrusion, continental underplating and lithospheric rifting. This study was undertaken to elucidate the geographic distribution of $^3He/^4He$ ratios around seismically active regions in Japan, using helium isotope data obtained from gas samples. Several case studies suggest that there seem to be a significant trend of high ^3He emanations around the source regions following inland earthquakes, resulting in leakage of mantle volatiles through crustal pathways (faults) due to more frequent development of higher permeability pathways and/or upwelling of mantle fluids through the ductile lower crust. The other case is significant decrease of $^3He/^4He$ ratios found in groundwaters before and after a large inland earthquake. Episodic faulting could release accumulated crustal (radiogenic) helium from host rocks, or enhance the transfer of mantle volatiles through permeable fault zones, such that subsequent fluid flow proximal to the source region could then explain the spatio-temporal variations in $^3He/^4He$ ratios.

---

* Corresponding author's e-mail : umeda.koji@jaea.go.jp.

In: Chemistry Research Summaries Volume 12
Editor: Lucille Monaco Cacioppo

ISBN: 978-1-61668-757-1
© 2014 Nova Science Publishers, Inc.

Chapter 101

WEAK SUPERFLUIDITY: NONSTATIONARY JOSEPHSON EFFECT IN He-4 AND POSSIBLE APPLICATIONS

A. M. Tskhovrebov and L. N. Zherikhina[*]
P. N. Lebedev Physical Institute of the Russian Academy of Sciences,
Moscow, Russia

RESEARCH SUMMARY

Unusual occurrences of nonstationary Josephson effect in superfluid He-4 are considered. Nonstationary Josephson effect is analyzed in the context with parametric amplifying of acoustic oscillations on kinetic nonlinearity of superfluid Josephson element. Mechanism of quantum fluctuations compression, following parametric rating, is taken into account. Appearance of Josephson fluxon in superfluid medium parted by a wall with narrow channels serving as weak links is analyzed by analogy with Josephson vortexes in the case of weak superconductivity. Possible applications of the effects above are discussed. Parametric amplifying of acoustic oscillations on conditions of quantum fluctuations compression is proposed to be used for making a high frequency (f >> 1000 Hz) gravitational waves detector. In this case if one have in mind that the efficiency of gravitational waves generation by a quadrupole radiator is proportional to the sixth power of frequency it seems interesting to use such a detector in a gravitational analog of Hertz experiment. Since superfluid Josephson vortexes are of quantum nature, it may be possible to model entangled states, which underline the matter wave q-bit system.

[*] E-mail: zherikh@sci.lebedev.ru.

In: Chemistry Research Summaries Volume 12
Editor: Lucille Monaco Cacioppo

ISBN: 978-1-61668-757-1
© 2014 Nova Science Publishers, Inc.

Chapter 102

CLEAN ENERGY FROM HELIUM-3 FUELLED MUON-CATALYZED ANEUTRONIC FUSION

Cooroo Egan[*]

RESEARCH SUMMARY

Helium-3 is a stable isotope of helium, terrestrially scarce, but with an estimated 6.5×10^8 kg contained within the lunar regolith. Despite the difficulties inherent in commercial exploitation of these remote reserves, research progresses into its potential for use in fusion. It has now been posited that by employing existing and developing technologies, an energy efficient, helium-3 fuelled, muon-catalyzed fusion (μCF) reactor is able to be constructed. This reactor, which avoids the problems associated with maintenance of the extremely high temperatures normally required to catalyze fusion, is also aneutronic, offering total freedom from the need to deal with radioactive materials. The key processes of this radiation free, helium-3 powered μCF reactor are discussed, including a review of some of the technologies that are required, the issue of alpha-sticking in the reaction area, and the predicted muon-wave that simulations have suggested would partially negate the alpha-sticking while providing the primary agency for the predicted energy efficiency.

---

[*] E-mail address: cooroo@ozlawyer.com. Affiliations: None at time of writing

In: Chemistry Research Summaries Volume 12
Editor: Lucille Monaco Cacioppo

ISBN: 978-1-61668-757-1
© 2014 Nova Science Publishers, Inc.

Chapter 103

ROLE OF MITOCHONDRIA IN THE GENERATION OF REACTIVE OXYGEN SPECIES

Giorgio Lenaz[*]

Department of Biomedical and Neuro Motor Sciences,
Operative Unit of Biochemistry,
University of Bologna, Bologna, Italy

RESEARCH SUMMARY

The mitochondrial respiratory chain, specially Complexes I and III and perhaps Complex II, is considered the main origin of ROS (superoxide and hydrogen peroxide), but several other sources may be important for ROS generation, such as mitochondrial p66[Shc], monoamine oxidase, α-ketoglutarate dehydogenase, besides redox cycling of redox-active molecules. It is generally assumed that conditions of high membrane potential favouring reverse electron transfer are those maximizing ROS generation from Complex I, although this proposal has been challenged. Several conditions affecting the rate of electron transfer in the respiratory chain are able to enhance ROS generation; among these, the disruption of respiratory supercomplexes is an important factor to increase the production of ROS. Mitochondrial ROS are able to modify lipids, proteins, carbohydrates and nucleic acids in mitochondria and to activate/inactivate signalling pathways by oxidative modification of redox-active factors. Cells are endowed with several defence mechanisms including repair or removal of damaged molecules, and antioxidant systems, either enymatic or non-enzymatic. Oxidative stress is at the basis of ageing and many pathological disorders, such as ischemic diseases, neurodegenerative diseases, diabetes, and cancer, although the underlying mechanisms are not always completely understood.

[*] E-mail giorgio.lenaz@unibo.it.

In: Chemistry Research Summaries Volume 12
Editor: Lucille Monaco Cacioppo

ISBN: 978-1-61668-757-1
© 2014 Nova Science Publishers, Inc.

Chapter 104

PARTICIPATION OF REACTIVE OXYGEN SPECIES IN FORMATION OF INDUCED RESISTANCES OF PLANTS TO ABIOTIC STRESSORS

Yu. E. Kolupaev[*] and Yu. V. Karpets
V. V. Dokuchaev Kharkiv National Agrarian University,
Kharkiv, Ukraine

RESEARCH SUMMARY

The possible reasons of intensifying of generation of reactive oxygen species (ROS) in plants under the influence of abiotic stressors are considered. The characteristic of hydrogen peroxide and superoxide anion-radical as signal messengers is given. The data about the basic cellular compartments involved in formation and detoxication of ROS are analyzed. Participation of the ROS-generating enzyme systems (NADPH oxidase, peroxidase, oxalate oxidase) and components of antioxidative system in formation of redox-signals is characterized. Possible sensors of redox-signals in plant cells are described. Interaction between ROS and other signal messengers, in particular nitrogen oxide and calcium ions, at the reaction of plants to the influence of abiotic stressors is discussed. The role of ROS in the development of plants resistance to hyperthermia and osmotic shock after the preliminary hardening influence by certain stressors is analyzed on the example of results of own investigations. Concrete protective reactions of plants to the action of abiotic stressors in which induction the ROS take part are considered. Influence on plants of the exogenous physiologically active compounds inducing protective reactions at intermediary of ROS is described.

---

[*] E-mail: plant_biology@mail.ru.

In: Chemistry Research Summaries Volume 12
Editor: Lucille Monaco Cacioppo

ISBN: 978-1-61668-757-1
© 2014 Nova Science Publishers, Inc.

Chapter 105

REACTIVE OXYGEN SPECIES (ROS): FORMATION, PHYSIOLOGICAL ROLES AND AUTOIMMUNE DISEASES

*Dilip Shah[1,2] and Mei X. Wu[2,3]**

[1]Center for Translational Medicine, Thomas Jefferson University,
Philadelphia, Pennsylvania, US
[2]Wellman Center for Photomedicine and Department of Dermatology,
Massachusetts General Hospital (MGH), Harvard Medical School (HMS),
Boston, Massachusetts, US and
[3]Harvard-MIT Division of Health Sciences and Technology, Boston, Massachusetts, US

RESEARCH SUMMARY

Increased formation of free radicals and altered redox state are of fundamental importance in the pathogenesis of autoimmune diseases. Free radicals are mainly derived from oxygen (reactive oxygen species/ROS) and nitrogen (reactive nitrogen species/RNS) at mitochondria and cellular and endoplasmic reticulum membranes as physiological responses to a variety of internal and external stress. These free radicals are well recognized for their beneficial and deleterious roles in our body's defense system. ROS/RNS are beneficial at low/moderate concentrations via activation of redox-sensitive signaling pathways, phagocytosis of the infected cells, induction of mitogenic responses for wound healing, and clearance of abnormal or aging cells as a part of surveillance mechanism. Excessive production of free radicals causes oxidative stress that results in oxidization of lipids, proteins, and DNA, detrimental to the immune system. The current chapter will be focused on following areas: (i) sources and generation of ROS/RNS and their scavengers; (ii) their physiological functions; (iii) alteration of redox state and autoimmune diseases; and (iv) biomarkers of oxidative stress in the management of autoimmune diseases. Attention is

* Correspondence: Mei X. Wu, Wellman Center for Photomedicine, Edwards 222, Massachusetts General Hospital, 50 Blossom Street, Boston, MA 02114. e-mail: (mwu2@partners.org).

specifically focused on the ROS/RNS-linked pathogenesis of systemic lupus erythematosus (SLE) and rheumatoid arthritis (RA).

In: Chemistry Research Summaries Volume 12   ISBN: 978-1-61668-757-1
Editor: Lucille Monaco Cacioppo   © 2014 Nova Science Publishers, Inc.

Chapter 106

METAL OXIDE NANOPARTICLES AS A SOURCE FOR ROS: THEIR APPLICATION IN THE FABRICATION OF ANTIMICROBIAL TEXTILES

Anat Lipovsky, Ilana Perelstein, Nina Perkas,
Rachel Lubart and Aharon Gedanken
Department of Chemistry, Center for Advanced Materials and Nanotechnology,
Bar-Ilan University, Ramat-Gan, Israel

RESEARCH SUMMARY

Reactive Oxygen Species – ROS (such as $^{\cdot}OH$, $O_2^{\cdot-}$, H_2O_2, $^{\cdot}HO_2$ and singlet oxygen) are the key components for killing bacteria by macrophages, H_2O_2 is long being used as a house hold desenfectant. In rescent years, an increased research in the field of nanoparticles (NPs) and their applications as antimicrobial substances revealed that the formation of ROS plays a significant role in their activity toward pathogen destruction.

This chapter will review the sonochemical preparation of metal oxide (MO) nanoparticles, their subsequent deposition on textiles via the sonochemical method, and their antimicrobial activity. The chapter will describe a research that has concentrated on characterizing the ROS mediated antimicrobial activity of ZnO, CuO and other MO nanoparticles. The principle of the sonochemical embedding of the nanoparticles into surfaces in general and textiles in particular will be explained. Finally, the work on the sonochemical functionalization of textiles for creation of smart antimicrobial fabrics will be also reviewed.

In: Chemistry Research Summaries Volume 12
Editor: Lucille Monaco Cacioppo

ISBN: 978-1-61668-757-1
© 2014 Nova Science Publishers, Inc.

Chapter 107

REACTIVE OXYGEN SPECIES: POTENTIAL DOUBLE-EDGED SWORD

Deepa Khanna[1] and Monika Garg
Rajendera Institute of Technology and Sciences, Hayana, India

RESEARCH SUMMARY

Reactive oxygen species (ROS) are an unavoidable by-product of cellular metabolism, can produced by interaction of ionizing radiation with biological molecule, and dedicated enzymes in phagocytic cells (NADPH oxidase and myeloperoxidase) or as a result of an imbalance between radical-generating and radical-scavenging systems. Physiological role of ROS is as a messenger in normal cell signal transduction and cell cycling. For activation of transcription factors from cytokine-receptor interactions, ROS are utilized as signalling messengers. ROS is necessary to maturation and membrane fusion of spermatozoa and oocyte during fertilization. NADPH oxidase enzyme activation and NO,a potential vasodilator produce an effective immune response with the help of ROS. H_2O_2, a ROS species has been suggested as a regulater of mitogen-activated protein kinase (MAPK) and p53 which control signalling mechanism. Normal potential of ROS get converted into deleterious action with their overproduction. Myocardial Infarction, Atherosclerosis, Parkinson Disease, Alzheimer Disease, Autoimmune Diseases, Radiation Injury, Emphysema and Sunburn are disorders caused by excessive ROS. ROS associated damage is carried by hydrogen peroxide (H_2O_2) molecules, hypochlorite ions (HOCl), hydroxyl (OH•), nitric oxide (NO•) radical, superoxide ($O2•^-$), peroxyl (ROO•) free radicals, and lipid peroxyl (LOO•). Mitochondria are the foremost site for in vivo production of ROS. Free radical generation is a continous chain reaction which extensively involved in development of various complications. Free radicals react with all biological macromolecules (lipids, proteins, nucleic acids and carbohydrates) contributing oxidative stress and activation of apoptotic pathway. Oxygen metabolism in aerobic organisms inevitably generates ROS, especially in the reduction of oxygen by mitochondrial electron transfer system causing oxidative stress. Oxidative stress alter various

---

[1] Corresponding Author: Professor and Head, Department of Pharmacology; Cardiovascular Pharmacology Division; Institute of Pharmacy; Rajendra Institute of Technology and Sciences (RITS); Sirsa-125 055, India; Phone: 0091-9416850005; Email address: 7drdeepa@gmail.com.

mitochondrial function including calcium homeostasis and triggering of permeability transition pore (PTP) and leading to decrease in the mitochondrial membrane potential. Further, intracellular ROS also affect the mitochondria by activation of caspases with the rapid release of cytochrome c which ultimately cause apoptosis. Tumour necrosis factor (TNF-a), can induce ROS by interacting with TNF receptor (TNF-Rl), leading to apoptosis/ necrosis. ROS induce apoptosis effecting 'Guardian of the genome' p53. Cells have various enzymatic and non-enzymatic antioxidant defense mechanisms to overcum the harmful effect of ROS. These antioxidants include superoxide dismutase (SOD), catalase, glutathione reductase, glutathione peroxidase, alpha-tocopherol (vitamin E), uric acid and vitamin C. In this chapter the emphasis are made is to highlight the physiological roles, formation mechanisms, and common harmful effects of ROS.

In: Chemistry Research Summaries Volume 12
Editor: Lucille Monaco Cacioppo

ISBN: 978-1-61668-757-1
© 2014 Nova Science Publishers, Inc.

Chapter 108

Photocatalytic Water Purification: Synergistic Effect with Reactive Oxygen Species (ROS)

Tsuyoshi Ochiai[1,2,] and Akira Fujishima[1,2]*

[1]Photocatalyst Group, Kanagawa Academy of Science
and Technology, Takatsu-ku, Kawasaki, Kanagawa, Japan
[2]Photocatalysis International Research Center,
Tokyo University of Science, Noda, Chiba, Japan

Research Summary

Application of the strong oxidation ability of photo-excited TiO_2 for water purification has received growing attention. Most of the aqueous contaminants such as haloalkanes, aliphatic alcohols, carboxylic acids, aromatics, polymers, surfactants, pesticides, and dyes, can be mineralized at the surface of UV-excited TiO_2 photocatalysts. However, the quantum yields measured in photocatalytic water purification varied over the wide range of 0.1–10%, which was several times lower than those of photocatalytic air purification. The main problems are that UV penetration depth is strongly limited in colored wastewater and mass transfer rate coefficient in the wastewater is lower than it in air. One of the solutions of these problems is combination with other processes or technologies such as electrolysis, sonolysis, and advanced oxidation processes (AOPs). Especially the combination with AOPs is useful for decomposition of contaminants at relatively low cost. AOPs refer toa set of chemical treatment methods designed to remove organics in water by oxidation through reactions with reactive oxygen species (ROS) such as •OH. The combination of TiO_2 photocatalysis with the other AOPs could enhance generation of ROS by synergistic effect. This chapter reviews these insights with several reports about photocatalytic water purification. Our recent studies are also mentioned.

---

* Email: pg-ochiai@newkast.or.jp.

In: Chemistry Research Summaries Volume 12
Editor: Lucille Monaco Cacioppo

ISBN: 978-1-61668-757-1
© 2014 Nova Science Publishers, Inc.

OXIDATIVE STRESS ON NEURODEGENERATION: IMPLICATIONS IN ALZHEIMER'S AND PARKINSON'S DISEASES

Elena González-Burgos and M. Pilar Gómez-Serranillos[*]
Department of Pharmacology, Faculty of Pharmacy,
University Complutense of Madrid, Madrid, Spain

RESEARCH SUMMARY

Oxidative stress occurs when the generation of ROS exceeds the capacity of the antioxidant defense system to remove or neutralize them, and the normal cellular redox state is altered. Reactive oxygen species, produced from both intracellular and extracellular sources (i.e., environmental pollutants, irradiation, drugs, etc.), can cause direct oxidative injury to biological molecules such as lipids, proteins and DNA. The accumulated ROS damage constitutes a major contributing factor to the pathogenesis of several neurodegenerative diseases, including Alzheimer's and Parkinson's diseases; these common progressive disorders of the central nervous system affects currently about 36 million and 10 million of people worldwide, respectively. In Alzheimer's disease, one of the key mechanisms reported for the neurotoxicity of the amyloid-beta peptide (Aβ) involves the production of ion-mediated hydrogen peroxide. In Parkinson's disease, the abnormal oxidative desamination and autooxidation of dopamine lead to the generation in excess of ROS such as hydroxyl radical, superoxide anion and hydrogen peroxide. Biochemical markers of ROS including lipid peroxidation products (HNE, MDA), oxidized bases in DNA (8-hydroxyguanine) and signs of mitochondrial dysfunction, detected in post-mortem brains, support the association of oxidative stress and the origination and development of these two neurodegenerative diseases. In this chapter, an overview of the mechanism related to oxidative stress in neurodegeneration, the potential role of specific products of oxidative modification of cellular components for diagnosis and finally, the most promising therapeutic strategies are reported.

---

[*] E-mail: pserra@ucm.es.

In: Chemistry Research Summaries Volume 12
Editor: Lucille Monaco Cacioppo

ISBN: 978-1-61668-757-1
© 2014 Nova Science Publishers, Inc.

Chapter 110

THE INTERPLAY BETWEEN REACTIVE OXYGEN SPECIES AND GASEOUS MESSENGER MOLECULES IN PLANT RESPONSE TO ENVIRONMENTAL STRESSES

Meng Zhang[1], Yan-Feng Xue[1*], Yan-Jun Li[1], Fengxiang X. Han[2], Wei-Min Xu[1], Zhi-Qi Shi[1†] and Jian Chen[1‡*]*
[1]Institute of Food Quality and Safety,
Jiangsu Academy of Agricultural Sciences, Nanjing, China
[2]Department of Chemistry and Biochemistry,
Jackson State University, Jackson, Mississippi, US

RESEARCH SUMMARY

Reactive oxygen species (ROS) play important roles in plant response to environmental stresses. Recent studies suggest that several endogenous gaseous messenger molecules, such as nitric oxide (NO), carbon monoxide (CO), and hydrogen sulfide (H_2S), have emerged as vital regulators in plant stress responses. Interestingly, these gaseous messenger molecules extensively interplay with ROS in multiple intrinsic physiological processes in plant adaption under various environmental stimuli. In this chapter, we highlight the recent advanced studies focusing on the roles of the regulation of ROS by gaseous messengers in modulating plant toxicity or tolerance to both biotic and abiotic stresses. The crosstalk between ROS and the signaling cassette of gaseous messengers is discussed as well. In addition, we propose a new scenario involving the potential roles of ROS in the dynamic network mediated by gaseous messengers in plant response to environmental stresses.

---

[*] These authors contribute equally to this work.
[†] The correspondence may also be addressed to Zhi-Qi Shi. 50 Zhongling street, Nanjing 210014, China. Tel: +86-25-84391863; Fax: +86-25-84390422; E-mail: nytrpz@yahoo.cn.
[‡] To whom correspondence should be addressed. Jian Chen. 50 Zhongling street, Nanjing 210014, China. Tel: +86-25-84391863; Fax: +86-25-84390422; E-mail: jacksonchen206@gmail.com.

In: Chemistry Research Summaries Volume 12
Editor: Lucille Monaco Cacioppo

ISBN: 978-1-61668-757-1
© 2014 Nova Science Publishers, Inc.

Chapter 111

REACTIVE OXYGEN SPECIES IN NON-INVASIVE CANCER THERAPY

Hirotomo Shibaguchi[*]

Department of Biochemistry, Faculty of Medicine,
Fukuoka University, Japan

RESEARCH SUMMARY

Reactive oxygen species (ROS) are highly reactive and are able to oxidize and to damage the biogenic molecules such as lipid, protein, DNA and enzyme, and results in cell death by apoptosis and/or by necrosis in tissues and cells. This property of ROS has used and developed in non-invasive cancer therapy as photodynamic therapy (PDT) or sonodynamic therapy (SDT). The common feature of these non-invasive treatments is the generation of ROS by irradiating light or ultrasound after administrating a harmless sensitizer. The sensitizer raises from ground state to excite state by irradiating light or ultrasound, followed by generation of ROS that involves singlet oxygen, hydrogen peroxide, superoxide anion and hydroxyl radical. Although the relationship between the chemical structure of sensitizer and the kind of ROS which was generated after light or ultrasound exposure is still unclear, cell death occurs by apoptosis, by autophagy and/or by necrosis, depending on concentration and localization of the sensitizer, cell type and exposure time and strength. Recently, the novel sensitizers that indicate strong antitumor effect in PDT or SDT have been reported not only in an *in vitro* experimental model but also in an *in vivo* animal model. So far, apoptosis has been reported as main pathway of cell death in PDT and SDT due to mitochondria and DNA dysfunction by ROS generated after localizing and accumulating sensitizer in cytoplasm. Interestingly, in addition to apoptosis, it turned out that necrosis, that occurs by impairing cellular membrane after ROS production from sensitizer localizing outside of the cells, is expectable as more than enough curative effect in these non-invasive cancer therapy.

---

[*] To whom correspondence: Hirotomo Shibaguchi, Department of Biochemistry, Faculty of Medicine, Fukuoka University, 7-45-1 Nanakuma, Jonan-ku, Fukuoka 814-0180, Japan. TEL: +81-92-801-1011. FAX: +81-92-801-3600. E-mail: shiba-h@fukuoka-u.ac.jp.

In: Chemistry Research Summaries Volume 12
Editor: Lucille Monaco Cacioppo

ISBN: 978-1-61668-757-1
© 2014 Nova Science Publishers, Inc.

Chapter 112

OXIDATIVE STRESS IN THE LUNGS AND BLOOD INDUCED BY SMOKING AND EXERCISE

*Shunsuke Taito[1] and Hironobu Hamada[2],**

[1]Department of Clinical Support, Hiroshima University Hospital,
Hiroshima, Japan
[2]Department of Physical Analysis and Therapeutic Sciences,
Graduate School of Biomedical & Health Sciences,
Hiroshima University, Hiroshima, Japan

RESEARCH SUMMARY

Oxidative stress is produced by reactive oxygen species (ROS) and is regulated by the expression and activity of antioxidants. Cigarette smoke is a complex mixture of thousands of chemical compounds, ROS and other oxidants, and is associated with increased oxidative stress in the lungs and blood that can contribute to several diseases. Exercise also induces oxidative stress, with the extent of ROS generation dependent on exercise intensity and duration. Cigarette smoking increases oxidative stress in concert with exercise, and cigarette smokers are reported to have increased pulmonary and plasma oxidative stress responses to strenuous exercise compared to nonsmokers. This review summarizes smoking- and exercise-induced oxidative stresses and the increased oxidative stress produced by the combination of smoking and exercise.

---

* Corresponding: Hironobu Hamada, M.D., Ph.D., Department of Physical Analysis and Therapeutic Sciences, Graduate School of Biomedical and Health Sciences, Hiroshima University, 1-2-3 Kasumi, Minami-ku, Hiroshima 734-8551, Japan. TEL & FAX: +81-82-257-5420. E-mail: hirohamada@hiroshima-u.ac.jp.

In: Chemistry Research Summaries Volume 12
Editor: Lucille Monaco Cacioppo

ISBN: 978-1-61668-757-1
© 2014 Nova Science Publishers, Inc.

Chapter 113

PLANT SIGNALING NETWORKS INVOLVING REACTIVE OXYGEN SPECIES AND CA^{2+}

Takamitsu Kurusu,[1,2,3,*] *Sachie Kimura,*[2] *Yuichi Tada,*[1]
Hidetaka Kaya[2,4] *and Kazuyuki Kuchitsu*[2,3]

[1]School of Bioscience and Biotechnology, Tokyo
University of Technology, Hachioji, Tokyo, Japan
[2]Department of Applied Biological Science, Tokyo
University of Science, Noda, Chiba, Japan
[3]Research Institute for Science and Technology, Tokyo
University of Science, Noda, Chiba, Japan
[4]Department of Biological Science, Graduate School of
Science, The University of Tokyo, Bunkyo-ku, Tokyo, Japan

RESEARCH SUMMARY

Although reactive oxygen species (ROS) are highly toxic substances and are produced during aerobic respiration and photosynthesis, recent studies have demonstrated that ROS, such as superoxide anion (O_2^-) and hydrogen peroxide (H_2O_2), are deliberately produced as important signaling messengers playing key roles in regulating a broad range of physiological processes including cellular growth and development as well as adaptation to environmental changes in plants. Given the toxicity of ROS, the enzymatic ROS production needs to be tightly regulated both spatially and temporally. Respiratory burst oxidase homologues (Rboh) have been identified as ROS-producing NADPH oxidases, which act as key signaling nodes integrating multiple signal transduction pathways in plants. We here discuss the

* Corresponding author: Takamitsu Kurusu, Ph. D. School of Bioscience and Biotechnology, Tokyo University of Technology, 1404-1 Katakura, Hachioji, Tokyo 192-0982, Japan. Department of Applied Biological Science, Tokyo University of Science, 2641 Yamazaki, Noda, Chiba 278-8510, Japan. Research Institute for Science and Technology, Tokyo University of Science, 2641 Yamazaki, Noda, Chiba 278-8510, Japan. E-mail: kurusutkmt@stf.teu.ac.jp.

interrelationship among signaling pathways involving Ca^{2+}, protein phosphorylation and Rboh-mediated ROS production, as well as physiological roles of the signaling networks.

In: Chemistry Research Summaries Volume 12   ISBN: 978-1-61668-757-1
Editor: Lucille Monaco Cacioppo   © 2014 Nova Science Publishers, Inc.

Chapter 114

FREE RADICALS AND ROLE OF ANTIOXIDANT ENZYMES ON IONIZING RADIATION RESISTANCE IN *ZYGOPHYLLUM FABAGO*, *PHRAGMITES AUSTRALIS*, *ARGUSIA SIBIRICA* L. AND *ELEAGNUS CASPICA* PLANTS

I. M. Huseynova*, K. H. Bayramova,
S. Y. Suleymanov and J. A. Aliyev
Institute of Botany, Azerbaijan National Academy of Sciences,
Baku, Azerbaijan

RESEARCH SUMMARY

Exposure all living organisms to ionizing radiation causes damage to tissue and can result in mutation, radiation sickness, cancer and death. Plant irradiation, induce oxidative stress with overproduction of reactive oxygen species (ROS) such as superoxide radicals ($O_2^{\bullet-}$), hydroxyl radicals (OH^-) and hydrogen peroxide (H_2O_2), which react rapidly with almost all structural and functional organic molecular, including proteins, lipids and nucleic asids causing disturbance of cellular metobalism. Histochemical analysis of accumulation of active species of oxygen has been carried out in plants (*Zygophyllum fabago*, *Phragmites australis*, *Argusia Sibirica L.*, *Eleagnus caspica*) exposed to 250 µR/hr radiation and in control plants. Significantly differences has been observed in the plant leafs exposed to radiation compared to the control due to the accumulation of superoxide radicals ($O_2^{\bullet-}$) and hydrogen peroxide (H_2O_2) in *Zygophyllum. fabago*. In *Phragmites australis* plants differences are less visible between control and stress leaves. Peroxide radicals was significantly detected in stressed leaves of *Argusia Sibirica L.* and *Eleagnus caspica* plants with comparison to healthy leaves. In *Zygophyllum fabago*, *Phragmites australis*, *Argusia Sibirica L.* plants exposed to ionizing radiation activity of catalase, has significantly increased in comparison with control plants,

*Corresponding author: Tel: +99412 5381164; Fax: +99412 5102433; E-mail: i_guseinova@mail.ru.

but its activity decreased (approximately 3.5 times) in *Eleagnus caspica*. APOX activity increased in *Eleagnus caspica* under the effect 250 μR/hr radiation. However contrary to the CAT, activity of APOX has decreased in stressed plants of *Zygophyllum fabago* and *Argusia Sibirica L.* compared with plants growing under the normal conditions. Electrophoretic spectrum of catalase was revealed only one high molecular weight isozyme (CAT 1) in plants having the impact of 250μR/hr background radiation and in control plants. High-intensity CAT 1 band was observed in *Phragmites australis*. Electrophoretic analysis of isozyme pattern of ascorbatperoxsidase in *Phragmites australis* was determined 5 isoforms in control and 6 isophorms of APOX in the radiation subjected plants. One isoform of APOX has newly appeared in stressed plants. Superoxidedismutase activity (SOD) dramatically increased in *Zygophyllum fabago* and *Argusia Sibirica L.* under the effects of radiation.

In: Chemistry Research Summaries Volume 12　　　　　ISBN: 978-1-61668-757-1
Editor: Lucille Monaco Cacioppo　　　　　© 2014 Nova Science Publishers, Inc.

Chapter 115

REACTIVE OXYGEN SPECIES AND WOUND HEALING

*Simona Martinotti, Bruno Burlando and Elia Ranzato**
DiSIT - Dipartimento di Scienze e Innovazione Tecnologica,
Università del Piemonte Orientale "Amedeo Avogadro",
Alessandria, Italy

RESEARCH SUMMARY

An injury may disturb the integrity of a tissue and thus inevitably results in a wound. The disturbed equilibrium of the local environment induces wound healing mechanisms. The wound healing process requires a fine balance between positive and deleterious effects exerted by reactive oxygen species (ROS), a group of extremely reactive molecules that are rate limiting in tissue regeneration. Understanding the role of ROS within a tissue will greatly enhance the possibility of manipulating wound healing. This chapter provides an overview on the role of ROS in wound repair and chronic wound pathogenesis.

──────────
* E-mail: ranzato@unipmn.it

In: Chemistry Research Summaries Volume 12
Editor: Lucille Monaco Cacioppo

ISBN: 978-1-61668-757-1
© 2014 Nova Science Publishers, Inc.

Chapter 116

GENDER DIMORPHISM IN HEPATIC OXIDATIVE STRESS INDUCED BY PROTEIN MALNUTRITION DURING PREGNANCY AND CHILDHOOD

Enrique Podaza, Tamara Vico,
*Stella Maris Echarte and Andrea Chisari**

Instituto de Investigaciones Biológicas,
Facultad de Ciencias Exactas y Naturales,
Universidad Nacional de Mar del Plata—CONICET,
Mar del Plata, Argentina

RESEARCH SUMMARY

Clinically, malnourished infants have increased markers of the metabolic syndrome by adolescence. Similarly, experimental rodent models with low birth weight are associated with hypertension, obesity, high cholesterol, insulin resistance and reduced longevity. Females show lower incidences of several metabolic diseases related to oxidative stress and mitochondrial dysfunction than males. Oxidative stress has been implicated in a large number of human diseases; altered homeostasis for ROS is one essential process that fundamentally contributes to mammalian vulnerability to sex-related diseases. Gender is a profound determinant factor of disease susceptibility and lifespan. Little is known about gender differences in oxidative homeostasis.

This review examines the evidence of the metabolic disease process involving the liver and oxidative stress induced by protein malnutrition in pregnant and lactating mothers, manifested in the adult lives of their offspring. Protein malnutrition in pregnant mothers induced changes in the oxidative status of livers of their offspring with marked sexual dimorphism. The content of reactive oxygen species, protein carbonylation and lipid peroxidation in liver cytosol were higher in males compared to females, although the total antioxidant capacity in males is higher than females. The study also highlights the complex

---

* Corresponding author's email: achisari@mdp.edu.ar.

nature of the injury of malnutrition in which the oxidation state correlates with the hepatic injury in a cause-and-effect manner, being higher in males than in females. An understanding of the reasons for this difference may help us to decrease the susceptibility to metabolic diseases of males and to understand the basic phenomenon of ageing, and to search for safe ways to increase the life span of males. Further elucidation of precise mechanisms responsible for the gender-related differences in the hepatic pathophysiology is essential for the potential clinical application of sex hormone modulation therapy.

In: Chemistry Research Summaries Volume 12
Editor: Lucille Monaco Cacioppo

ISBN: 978-1-61668-757-1
© 2014 Nova Science Publishers, Inc.

Chapter 117

HYDROPHILIC INTERACTION LIQUID CHROMATOGRAPHY: FUNDAMENTALS AND APPLICATIONS

Yuegang Zuo[1,], Si Zhou[1], Ruiting Zuo[2], Tian Shi[1], Yang Yang[1] and Patricia Henegan[1]*

[1]Department of Chemistry and Biochemistry, University of Massachusetts Dartmouth, North Dartmouth, Massachusetts, US
[2]Novi High School, Novi, Michigan, US

RESEARCH SUMMARY

Hydrophilic interaction liquid chromatography (HILIC) is an effective alternative to conventional HPLC techniques for the separation and determination of polar and hydrophilic compounds. Since Alpert described it first in 1990, the popularity of HILIC has been growing exponentially as measured by the number of publications due to an increasing demand for the analysis of polar components in complex matrices. HILIC is a chromatographic technique that uses aqueous-organic solvent mobile phases with a high percentage of organic solvent, and a polar stationary phase. So far, silica gels, amino, amide, cyano, carbamate-, diol- and zwitterionic-based stationary phases have been utilized in HILIC separation. Like other HPLC techniques, the understanding of HILIC retention mechanisms and theories has been behind the practice. In this chapter, we will discuss the development, basic separation mechanisms, stationary and mobile phases of HILIC, and summarize the applications of HILIC in several research fields such as bioanalysis, metabolomics, food, pharmaceutical, forensic and environmental sciences.

---

[*] Corresponding Author address: Department of Chemistry and Biochemistry, University of Massachusetts Dartmouth, 285 Old Westport Road, North Dartmouth, MA 02747, USA. Email: yzuo@umassd.edu, Phone: 508-999-8959, Fax: 508-999-9167.

In: Chemistry Research Summaries Volume 12
Editor: Lucille Monaco Cacioppo

ISBN: 978-1-61668-757-1
© 2014 Nova Science Publishers, Inc.

Chapter 118

THE NEW GENERATION OF HPLC COLUMNS: EVOLUTION OF PACKING MATERIALS

*Victoria Samanidou** and Chrysa Nazyropoulou*

Laboratory of Analytical Chemistry, Department of Chemistry,
Aristotle University of Thessaloniki, Greece

RESEARCH SUMMARY

Fast and accurate analysis is a prerequisite in all analytical fields and achieving reliable results by low-budget instrumentation is highly appreciated. HPLC is the most widely applied separation technique with numerous applications, as it is considered to be the most useful tool for the accurate and precise determination of a wide range of analytes.

The most crucial factorin chromatographic separation is undoubtedly the quality of the column. In this chapter we present the advanced technology on packing materials currently used in chromatographic columns. Column technology evolution has recently lead to the manufacture of sub-2 μm particle size columns used for Ultra High Performance Chromatography. However, the use of these columns with conventional chromatographic systems (with a pressure limit of 400 bar) is restricted due to pressure limitations.

The latter can be overcome by using new systems, capable of withstanding higher pressures of 1000 bar, but the cost of these systems is high and sometimes restrictive for low-budget laboratories. On the other hand, solid core particles can lead to ultra high performance analysis using conventional HPLC instrument. This chapter presents new HPLC packing materials. Sub-2μm porous particles, solid core particles and monolithic columns are compared to conventional columns in terms of efficiency, speed, resolution (as given by chromatographic equations) and comparative applications. The future in column technology is further discussed.

---

* Corresponding Author address: Laboratory of Analytical Chemistry, Department of Chemistry, Aristotle University of Thessaloniki, Greece, Tel: +302310997698, Fax: +302310997719. Email: samanidu@chem.auth.gr.

In: Chemistry Research Summaries Volume 12   ISBN: 978-1-61668-757-1
Editor: Lucille Monaco Cacioppo   © 2014 Nova Science Publishers, Inc.

Chapter 119

HIGH-PERFORMANCE LIQUID CHROMATOGRAPHY FOR CARBOHYDRATE ANALYSIS

*Xun Yan**

Analytical Sciences, Research & Development,
Amway Corporation, Michigan, US

RESEARCH SUMMARY

Carbohydrates are widely present in biological systems in both free states (e.g., starch, cellulose) and conjugated forms (e.g., proteoglycans, glycoproteins, glycolipids), providing energy storage as well as structural support functions. Carbohydrates participate in many biological processes including cell recognition, development, interaction, and inflammation. The analysis of carbohydrates is challenging due to their complex structure and heterogeneity. This chapter reviews current high-performance liquid chromatography (HPLC) techniques for carbohydrate analysis.

To analyze carbohydrate content by HPLC, the test sample must first be extracted and purified. Hydrolysis and derivatization techniques are used to release and label carbohydrates for sensitive and selective detection. There are several operational modes of HPLC that are widely used for carbohydrate separation including, reversed phase (RP) and normal phase (NP) chromatography, hydrophobic interaction chromatography (HIC), hydrophilic interaction liquid chromatography (HILIC), anion exchange chromatography (AEC), and size exclusion chromatography (SEC). Common detection methods used for HPLC include refractive index (RI), ultraviolet and visible (UV-Vis) absorbance, fluorescence, evaporative or laser light scattering (ELS or LLS), and electrochemical (EC) detection.

To demonstrate an HPLC application for analyzing carbohydrates, we have included a chitosan analysis method in this chapter. Chitosan, is a copolymer of glucosamine (2-amido-2-deoxy-D-glucose) and N-acetyl glucosamine via a β(1-4) linkage. It is a widely used food ingredient and additive. To quantify chitosan, it is first hydrolyzed to glucosamine with hydrochloric acid (HCl), and then undergoes derivatization with

---

* Corresponding Author 7575 Fulton Street E., Ada, MI, 49355, Email: xun.yan@amway.com.

N-(9-fluorenylmethoxycarbonyloxy)succinimide (FMOC-OSu). The glucosamine-FMOC derivatives are then separated and quantified using reversed phase HPLC with UV detection.

In: Chemistry Research Summaries Volume 12   ISBN: 978-1-61668-757-1
Editor: Lucille Monaco Cacioppo   © 2014 Nova Science Publishers, Inc.

Chapter 120

HIGH-PERFORMANCE LIQUID CHROMATOGRAPHY FOR THE ANALYSIS OF NON-NUCLEOSIDE REVERSE TRANSCRIPTASE INHIBITORS IN BIOLOGICAL FLUIDS AND PHARMACEUTICAL PRODUCTS

*Virginia Melis, Iris Usach and José-Esteban Peris**
Department of Pharmacy and Pharmaceutical Technology,
Faculty of Pharmacy, University of Valencia, Valencia, Spain

RESEARCH SUMMARY

Infections with the human immunodeficiency virus (HIV) are typically treated with drug combinations consisting of at least three different antiretroviral drugs. A drug belonging to the group of non-nucleoside reverse transcriptase inhibitors (NNRTIs) is an essential component of this highly active antiretroviral therapy (HAART). NNRTIs are orally administered and subjected to large interindividual, and sometimes intraindividual, variability in their plasma levels, which sustains the convenience of drug plasma concentration monitoring to enhance the outcome of antiretroviral therapy. In this regard, high performance liquid chromatography (HPLC) constitutes a rapid, specific and sensitive technique for determining NNRTI plasma concentrations in routine clinical practice. HPLC is also commonly used for the quality control tests of pharmaceutical products containing NNRTIs and for evaluating the purity of the active substance. This chapter reviews the use of HPLC for the analysis of non-nucleoside reverse transcriptase inhibitors. In particular, sample preparation, chromatographic conditions and detection methods are reported for biological fluids and pharmaceutical products.

* Corresponding Author: jose.e.peris@uv.es.

In: Chemistry Research Summaries Volume 12
Editor: Lucille Monaco Cacioppo

ISBN: 978-1-61668-757-1
© 2014 Nova Science Publishers, Inc.

Chapter 121

HIGH-PERFORMANCE LIQUID CHROMATOGRAPHY – AN EFFECTIVE TOOL FOR QUALITY CONTROL OF NATURAL CHOLESTEROL-LOWERING AGENTS

Ana Mornar, Miranda Sertić and Biljana Nigović*
Faculty of Pharmacy and Biochemistry University of Zagreb, Zagreb, Croatia

RESEARCH SUMMARY

Hyperlipidemia is a heterogeneous group of disorders characterized by an excess of lipids in the bloodstream. Regardless of the cause, it is a major modifiable risk factor for artherosclerosis or coronary artery disease. The most commonly used medication for the treatment of high cholesterol levels are statins such as atorvastatin, simvastatin and lovastatin. Although safe and effective, statins can cause muscle problems, lung and liver disorders as well as kidney damage. Therefore, many patients seek alternative therapies to control their cholesterol levels. Many natural cholesterol-lowering agents are widely available to the public as dietary supplements. A dietary supplement, also known as a food supplement, is a preparation intended to supplement the diet and provide nutrients. Dietary supplements are usually used by patients at their own discretion, in an unmonitored setting and without the input of their physicians. Dietary supplements are readily available, not classified as over-the-counter medications, and not regulated as such. Health practitioners and patients often consider these products safe and probably effective. Unfortunately, information on dietary supplements in nonmedical literature and even in scientific literature is usually unreliable. Moreover, numerous studies have used products that were not well characterized. There is no uniform legislation in the dietary supplements area despite their ever growing popularity and presence on the market. Health safety, nutritional value and laboratory control of declared content is very rare. Therefore, greater attention has recently been given to quality control of dietary supplements. Today advance analytical techniques can be employed for identification and quantification of active compounds as well as toxic ingredients in dietary supplements. Due to its superior precision, high resolution and capacity to analyze thermally labile and

---

* Corresponding author: Email: amornar@pharma.hr.

non-volatile compounds, high-performance liquid chromatography is applied for the quality control of dietary supplements. In this chapter a critical review on chromatographic methods for quality control of most frequently used natural cholesterol-lowering dietary supplements such as red fermented rice, artichoke, phytosterols, omega-3 fatty acids, green tea, soybean, gugulipid, coenzyme Q_{10}, taurine, flax seeds and policosanol is given. Special attention is paid to determination of active ingredients as well as toxic compounds. Additionally, sample preparation procedures and chromatographic methods used for determination of active ingredients in biological fluids are discussed.

In: Chemistry Research Summaries Volume 12   ISBN: 978-1-61668-757-1
Editor: Lucille Monaco Cacioppo   © 2014 Nova Science Publishers, Inc.

Chapter 122

MEASUREMENT OF CHOLESTEROL LEVELS OF LIPOPROTEIN CLASSES BY USING ANION-EXCHANGE CHROMATOGRAPHY

Yuji Hirowatari[1], Hidekatsu Yanai[2] and Hiroshi Yohida[3]

[1]Bioscience Division, TOSOH CORPORATION, Japan
[2]Department of Internal Medicine, National Center for Global Health
and Medicine, Kohnodai Hospital, Chiba, Japan
[3]Department of Laboratory Medicine, Jikei University Kashiwa Hospital,
Chiba, Japan

RESEARCH SUMMARY

The relationship between lipoprotein profile in blood and progress of atherosclerosis is investigated in a lot of studies. A low cholesterol level of high-density lipoprotein (HDL), and high cholesterol levels of low-density lipoprotein (LDL), intermediate-density lipoprotein (IDL), and very-low-density lipoprotein (VLDL) are well known to be the risk markers for atherosclerotic disease such as coronary heart disease. The changes of lipoprotein levels are seen in patients with the impaired lipoprotein metabolism. Therefore, the development of the analysis method for estimation of lipoprotein profile is important for clinical diagnosis and medical care of the diseases.

The methods for analyzing lipoprotein profiles by using ultracentrifugation, electrophoresis, gel-permeation chromatography, and anion-exchange chromatography were previously reported. All major lipoprotein classes (HDL, LDL, IDL, VLDL, chylomicron, etc.) can be separated by ultracentrifugation which is a standard method for separation of lipoprotein classes, but it is laborious and time-consuming. HDL, LDL, and VLDL can be separated by electrophoresis and gel-permeation-chromatography, however, LDL and VLDL in patients with diabetes or hyperlipidemia sometimes cannot be separated precisely. We developed an anion-exchange high-performance liquid chromatographic (AEX-HPLC) method using a column containing diethylaminoethyl-ligand nonporous polymer-based gel with a step gradient of sodium perchlorate concentration, by which HDL, LDL, IDL, VLDL, chylomicron, and lipoprotein(a) can be separated, even in blood from the patients with diabetes or hyperlipidemia. Additionally, we reported that the subfractions in HDL and LDL in human blood and the major five lipoprotein classes (HDL, LDL, IDL, VLDL, and chylomicron) in rabbit blood can be separated by the AEX-HPLC method.

The AEX-HPLC method which has a high ability of separation of lipoprotein classes is suitable for the convenient and accurate assay of lipoprotein profile in clinical studies.

In: Chemistry Research Summaries Volume 12   ISBN: 978-1-61668-757-1
Editor: Lucille Monaco Cacioppo   © 2014 Nova Science Publishers, Inc.

Chapter 123

RECENT TRENDS IN LC ANALYSIS OF BIOLOGICAL MATERIALS FOR DETERMINATION OF BENZODIAZEPINE DRUGS

Karolina Persona and Katarzyna Madej[*]

Department of Analytical Chemistry, Faculty of Chemistry,
Jagiellonian University, Krakow, Poland

RESEARCH SUMMARY

Benzodiazepines belong to the most commonly self-administered group of sedative, antianxiety and anticonvulsant drugs. Generally, they are known as safe drugs because of their high therapeutic index. However, the use of these pharmaceuticals together with other drugs or substances (e.g., alcohol) may result in serious consequences. Some benzodiazepines (e.g., flunitrazepam) are used for criminal purposes as date rape drugs. Therefore, a variety of biological materials, both conventional (plasma, serum, urine) and alternative (hair, saliva, vitreous humor, nails), have been investigated for these medicines. In the last decade, liquid chromatographic methods, especially LC/MS(MS), have played a dominant role in the determination of benzodiazepine drugs in biological samples. Analysis of biological material by LC methods usually should be preceded by sample preparation using extraction techniques such as SPE, LLE or MAE. In this chapter, recent developments of LC methods for benzodiazepine determination, covering mostly the last five years in two of the main areas of pharmacological study and toxicological analysis, are presented and explained with the providing of their appropriate applications.

[*] Corresponding author: Jagiellonian University, Ingardena 3 Street, 30-060 Krakow, Poland. Email: madejk@chemia.uj.edu.pl, tel.: +48126635602; fax: +48126635600.

In: Chemistry Research Summaries Volume 12   ISBN: 978-1-61668-757-1
Editor: Lucille Monaco Cacioppo   © 2014 Nova Science Publishers, Inc.

Chapter 124

HPLC ANALYTICAL STUDY OF METHACRYLIC MONOMERS RELEASED FROM DENTAL COMPOSITE MATERIALS

Giuseppina Nocca[1], Virginia Carbone[2], Alessandro Lupi[3], Sandro Rengo[4] and Gianrico Spagnuolo[4]*

[1]Istituto di Biochimica e Biochimica Clinica,
Università Cattolica del Sacro Cuore, Roma, Italy
[2]Istituto di Scienze dell'Alimentazione, CNR, Avellino, Italy
[3]Istituto di Chimica del Riconoscimento Molecolare, CNR, Roma, Italy
[4]Dipartimento di Scienze Odontostomatologiche e Maxillofacciali, Università di Napoli
"Federico II", Napoli, Italy

RESEARCH SUMMARY

Triethylene glycol dimethacrylate (TEGDMA) and 2-hydroxyethyl methacrylate (HEMA) are methacrylic monomers present in dental auto- and photo-polymerizable resins. Many in vitro studies have shown that the polymerization of the above mentioned compounds is never complete and the uncured monomers are released in the oral environment, causing possible local adverse effects. The evaluation of the amounts of the methacrylic monomers released from composite resins is therefore very important and HPLC technique is particularly suitable to this purpose. HPLC is however not limited to qualitative and quantitative analysis of methacrylic monomers but can be also applied to the study of their metabolism. The present work summarizes the recent results about the detection of TEGDMA and HEMA in complex systems like cells and culture media by HPLC, evidencing its key role in the investigations of the substances involved in cytotoxic processes. Moreover the great specificity and sensibility of the used method allow to relate the concentration values of

---

* Corresponding author: Giuseppina Nocca, Istituto di Biochimica e Biochimica Clinica, Università Cattolica del Sacro Cuore, Roma, Italy. Email: g.nocca@rm.unicatt.it.

methacrylic monomers to their cytotoxic effects, in particular when such molecules are used in presence of N-acetyl cysteine, helping to clarify its mechanism of detoxification.

In: Chemistry Research Summaries Volume 12
Editor: Lucille Monaco Cacioppo

ISBN: 978-1-61668-757-1
© 2014 Nova Science Publishers, Inc.

Chapter 125

HPLC ANALYSIS OF VITAMIN B_1, B_2, B_3, B_6, B_9, B_{12} AND VITAMIN C IN VARIOUS FOOD MATRICES

Jessy van Wyk[1], Larry Dolley[2] and Ndumiso Mshicileli[2]*

[1]Department of Food Technology, Cape Peninsula University of Technology,
Bellville, South Africa
[2]Agrifood Technology Station, Cape Peninsula University of Technology,
Bellville, South Africa

RESEARCH SUMMARY

Various methods had been described for the analysis of vitamins in food matrices, with more and more of these including the use of HPLC to measure the levels of these micronutrients in foodstuffs. The renewed interest in rapid and accurate quantification of micronutrients in foodstuffs is due to more stringent requirements by food regulatory agencies around the world. Legislation now demands that the nutrition information displayed on food labels be backed up by reliable results obtained using validated analyses. Three challenges are common in terms of quantifying vitamins in food matrices: 1) extraction techniques that are sufficiently effective to liberate the various forms of the vitamin from each unique matrix, 2) ensuring that labile forms of the vitamin are protected against degeneration by light and/or air (oxygen) for a sufficiently long period to afford accurate quantification and 3) obtaining an analytical method with sufficient sensitivity, selectivity, accuracy and precision, with cost and time also being considerations. The chapter dealt with these aspects concerning vitamin B_1, B_2, B_3, B_6, B_9, B_{12} and vitamin C. Extraction procedures were described, as well as typical HPLC methods and recent improvements in this field.

* Corresponding author: Email: vanwykj@cput.ac.za.

In: Chemistry Research Summaries Volume 12   ISBN: 978-1-61668-757-1
Editor: Lucille Monaco Cacioppo   © 2014 Nova Science Publishers, Inc.

Chapter 126

Ultra Performance Liquid Chromatography Coupled to Ultraviolet-Vis and Mass Spectrometry Detector for Screening of Organic Acids and Polyphenols in Red Wine

M. Gonzalez-Hernandez[1,2]*, J. M. Avizcuri-Inac[2,3],
M. Dizy[1,2] and P. Fernández-Zurbano[2,3]
[1]Departamento de Agricultura y Alimentación, La Rioja, Spain
[2]Instituto de Ciencias de Vid y el Vino (UR-CSIC-GR), La Rioja, Spain
[3]Departamento de Química, University of La Rioja, La Rioja, Spain

RESEARCH SUMMARY

This chapter describes the development and optimization of three chromatographic methods based on ultra-performance liquid chromatography (UPLC) coupled to electrospray ionization (ESI) – tandem mass spectrometry (MS/MS) and ultraviolet visible (UV-vis) detectors for the identification and quantification of seven organic acids (*trans*-aconitic acid, *cis*-aconitic acid, tartaric acid, succinic acid, L(+)-lactic acid, L(-)-malic acid and citric acid) and sixty-four wine polyphenols of which five were hydroxybenzoic acid and derivatives, eight hydroxycinamic acid and derivatives, two stilbenes, nine flavan-3-ols, twelve flavonols and twenty-six anthocyanins. The identification and quantification of organic acids in wine was performed using the UPLC-ESI-MS/MS under isocratic conditions and with the electrospray ionization source operating in negative mode. A second method was developed for the determination of *cis/trans* aconitic acid and non-pigmented polyphenols, while UPLC was accomplished using ESI-MS/MS and UV-vis detectors. Finally, UPLC coupled to ESI-MS/MS and UV-vis detection results in effective and fast screening of the anthocyanin pigments. Separation was achieved with an Acquity BEH C_{18} (100 mm x 2.1 mm, 1.7 µm) column. The relative standard deviation (RSD) for the repeatability test (n=5) of peak area

---

* Corresponding author: Email: marivelgh@gmail.com.

and retention time were all below 1.47% and 0.03% for ESI-MS/MS and UV-vis detection respectively. A good separation of organic acids and phenolic compounds was achieved in 12.5 min. The applicability of this analytical approach was confirmed by the successful analysis of red wine samples.

In: Chemistry Research Summaries Volume 12
Editor: Lucille Monaco Cacioppo

ISBN: 978-1-61668-757-1
© 2014 Nova Science Publishers, Inc.

Chapter 127

HPLC–UV-Vis–ESI MS Examination of Archeological Fibers: Red Natural Dyes in Italian Textiles from 15th and 16th Centuries

Katarzyna Lech and Maciej Jarosz[*]
Warsaw University of Technology, Faculty of Chemistry, Warsaw, Poland

RESEARCH SUMMARY

High performance liquid chromatography (HPLC) coupled with spectrophotometric (UV-Vis) and electrospray mass spectrometric (MS) detection was applied to examination of natural colorants used for dyeing of historical textiles. Five examined red fibers were taken from Italian velvet brocades (parts of chasubles) dated at the 15th and 16th century, belonging to the collection of the Wawel Cathedral treasury (Cracow, Poland). In extracts from these fibers carminic, kermesic, flavokermesic and laccaic acids, alizarin, purpurin and munjistin were found. Successful identification of natural preparations used for dyeing examined textiles: dyes of animal origin – lac dye, Polish and Mexican cochineal, and also produced from plants – various madder species, confirmed unique potential of liquid chromatography in analyses of objects of historical value.

---

[*] Corresponding author: Email: mj@ch.pw.edu.pl.

In: Chemistry Research Summaries Volume 12
Editor: Lucille Monaco Cacioppo

ISBN: 978-1-61668-757-1
© 2014 Nova Science Publishers, Inc.

Chapter 128

CLAYS AS SUSTAINABLE CATALYSTS FOR ORGANIC TRANSFORMATIONS

B. S. Jai Prakash[1], Y. S. Bhat[2] and C. Ravindra Reddy[3]

[1]Department of Materials Sciences, Poornaprajna Institute
of Scientific Research, Bidalur Post, Devanahalli, Bangalore, India
[2]Department of Chemistry, Bangalore Institute of Technology, Bangalore, India
[3]Department of Chemical Engineering, University of Waterloo,
Waterloo, Ontario, Canada

RESEARCH SUMMARY

Catalysis is one of the important tools for sustainability and profitability of chemical production processes. The total quantity of catalysts used all over the world in all the processes together exceeds several million tonnes per annum. Their handling during use in the chemical transformation and disposal after use is of great environment concern. Many heterogeneous catalysts used for organic transformations are either toxic or non-specific or involve cumbersome procedures for their preparation and require a specialized care for their use, recovery and disposal which make the manufacturing process more and more energy intensive. There is obviously a continuous search for green catalysts which play a critical role in industrial reactions. An ideal green catalyst is a non-hazardous substance that can bring about a reaction at a faster rate and at lower temperatures than in the homogeneous conditions, yield maximum desired product with minimum waste, and which can be easily separated and recovered to be used more than once. Conventional heterogeneous catalysts such as metals, metal oxides, solid acids, low-dimensional solids and ion exchange resins are being used extensively in organic synthesis. Although very few of these fit into the definition of an ideal green catalyst, in the recent years there has been resurgence in the study of these catalysts, with or without modifications, reporting improved product yield and selectivity and reuse of the catalyst claiming green nature of the reaction.

A recent trend in the chemical industry is to switch over to catalysts that are more benign to environment. Advantages associated with this are easy handling of the catalysts during life cycle and disposal after use. In this context one such material that is being tried in variety of reactions is the clay based material. Clays may be regarded as green catalytic materials as they are abundantly available in nature and can be used with minimum processing. They are non-corrosive solid materials, have plasticity for easy fabrication into desired shape and size for use in the reactor, could easily be separated from product stream, are disposable relatively easily after use with no threat to ambience. Among the clays, the most used catalysts in chemical transformations are the montmorillonites.

Several options for the surface modification of montmorillonite practiced by clay chemists are available. These include (i) ion exchange with multivalent inorganic cations and coordination complexes to incorporate red-ox species and simultaneously generating acid centres (ii) ion exchange with organic cationic species having long alkyl chains with bulky head groups and intercalation with organic compounds to swell the clay layers to variable extents (iii) treatment with inorganic hydroxyl-oligomeric species followed by thermal treatment to obtain pillared clays having Lewis acidity (iv) treatment with mineral and organic acids and surfactants to get acid clays with tunable porosities (v) dealumination of structural aluminum by mild acid treatment to generate porosity in the clay platelets as well as mixed Brønsted acids in the interlayer (vi) incorporation of polymeric hydrated species of metals along with alkylamine species In the interlayer followed by removal of the organic species by washing with organic solvents and thermal treatment to get porous clay heterostructures (vii) impregnation of metal salts followed by reduction to get supported metal and metal oxide catalysts and (vii) modification for microwave-assisted reactions as clays with their variety of bipolarity are excellent absorbers of microwaves. All these are simple methods of surface modification making use of non-hazardous chemicals. Modified clays are invariably stable and do not lose their characteristics easily.

There have been a number of reviews on the modification of clays in the recent years. Hundreds of publications are appearing every year on their applications in organic synthesis. Some of the reviews which have appeared recently have presented the ability of clay catalysts to bring about organic transformations such as addition, condensation, alkylation, rearrangement, isomerization, cyclization, ring-opening and closure, oxidation, hydrogenation and dehydrogenation, protection-deprotection, hydroboration and so on. But the reviewers have disregarded the role played by the modified surface. They do not relate the changed features of the modified clay surface with the performance characteristics. The objective of this chapter is to review publications appeared on clay catalysis in the recent years with a view to present to the readers a detailed discussion on the various techniques of chemical modification with particular emphasis on their utility as green catalysts.

In: Chemistry Research Summaries Volume 12
Editor: Lucille Monaco Cacioppo

ISBN: 978-1-61668-757-1
© 2014 Nova Science Publishers, Inc.

Chapter 129

SOLVENT SELECTION FOR GREEN CHEMISTRY

Adi Wolfson and Dorith Tavor

Green Processes Center, Chemical Engineering Department,
Sami Shamoon College of Engineering, Beer-Sheva, Israel

RESEARCH SUMMARY

Solvent selection plays a key role in promoting sustainable chemical processes. The use of green solvents that allow substrate and catalyst dissolution, increase reaction activity and selectivity, and facilitate product separation and catalyst recycling is advantageous. A variety of environmentally friendly solvents, such as water, ionic liquids, and glycerol, can be used, and matching between reaction requirements and solvent nature should be considered.

In: Chemistry Research Summaries Volume 12
Editor: Lucille Monaco Cacioppo

ISBN: 978-1-61668-757-1
© 2014 Nova Science Publishers, Inc.

Chapter 130

LIGHT-DRIVEN CATALYSIS

María González-Béjar[1,2]*, Julia Pérez-Prieto[2],
and Juan Cesar Scaiano[1]

[1]Department of Chemistry and Centre for Catalysis Research and Innovation,
University of Ottawa, Ottawa, Ontario, Canada
[2]Instituto de Ciencia Molecular/ICMOL, Universidad de Valencia,
Valencia, Spain

RESEARCH SUMMARY

There is no doubt that light is the greenest reagent for catalytic processes. In this chapter the use of organic molecules, organometallic complexes, semiconductors and metallic nanoparticles in catalytic processes driven by light is discussed. Basic photochemistry concepts are highlighted in each example. Light-driven processes are used in many applications, such as water splitting, photovoltaics, hydrogen production, organic synthesis... This chapter is not meant to be an extensive review of possible photocatalyzed processes, but even so, it will let the reader design greener photocatalytic processes to create new chemical bonds using different illumination sources.

---
* Author Email Address: maria.gonzalez@uv.es. Fax: (+)1 613 562 5633.

In: Chemistry Research Summaries Volume 12
Editor: Lucille Monaco Cacioppo

ISBN: 978-1-61668-757-1
© 2014 Nova Science Publishers, Inc.

Chapter 131

PROGRESS IN SOLVENT-FREE SONOCHEMICAL ASSISTED SYNTHESIS OF FINE AND SPECIALTY CHEMICALS

V. Calvino-Casilda

Catalytic Spectroscopic Laboratory, Institute of Catalysis
and Petrochemistry, CSIC, Madrid, Spain

RESEARCH SUMMARY

Sonochemistry is an efficient non-classical method of activation in synthetic chemistry employed for decades with varied success. In recent years, ultrasonic energy has been presented as an alternative tool to prepare fine and specialty chemicals under mild conditions in order to minimize both production cost and waste generation.

The effects of ultrasound observed during organic reactions are due to cavitation, a physical process that creates, enlarges, and implodes gaseous and vaporous cavities in an irradiated liquid. Cavitation induces very high local temperatures and pressures inside the bubbles (cavities), leading to turbulent flow of the liquid and enhanced mass transfer. This high-energy input is known to induce new reactivities leading to the formation of unexpected chemical species and enhancing mechanical effects in heterogeneous processes. Thus, the remarkable phenomenon of cavitation makes sonochemistry unique even in solvent-free conditions preventing the production of large quantities of wastes in both fine and specialty chemicals industries. It is evident that nowadays continued progress in ultrasound-assisted organic synthesis facilitates and inspires future research in the field of sonochemistry.

In: Chemistry Research Summaries Volume 12
Editor: Lucille Monaco Cacioppo

ISBN: 978-1-61668-757-1
© 2014 Nova Science Publishers, Inc.

Chapter 132

HEAVY METALS, SYNTHETIC DYES, AND INDUSTRIAL OXIDATION REACTIONS: GREEN ALTERNATIVES FROM MATERIALS CHEMISTRY

Gustavo P. Ricci[1], Emerson H. de Faria[1], Liziane Marçal[1], Michelle Saltarelli[1], Paulo S. Calefi[1], Eduardo J. Nassar[1], and Katia J. Ciuffi[1]

[1]Universidade de Franca – Av. Dr. Armando Salles Oliveira,
Franca SP, Brasil

RESEARCH SUMMARY

Materials science is totally inserted in current developments in the areas of computing, electronics, engineering, medicine, pharmaceutics, energy, and industrial manufacture. Nowadays, it is one of the main green alternatives to reverse the environmental damage that these recent advances, unsustainable in their majority, have caused.

In this context, this chapter discusses the advances of materials chemistry in both the control of some industrial water pollutants (heavy metals and synthetic dyes) and the use of ecological and/or milder procedures in industrial oxidation processes.

Today, industrial wastewater is one of the most serious environmental problems. The inorganic and/or organic pollutants present in the wastes are generally originated due to negligent waste treatments or even no waste treatment at all. Heavy metals, especially Pb^{2+}, Cr^{6+}, Hg^{2+} and Cd^{2+}, commonly found in industrial effluents of leather tanning, pigments, and batteries industries, as well as mining are potential pollutants because of their toxic and lethal effects. Moreover, they are non-biodegradable and tend to accumulate in living organisms, thereby causing severe diseases. In turn, synthetic dyes, represented mainly by the azo-dyes employed in the textile industry, not only cause visual pollution of water bodies, but also diminish the photosynthetic activity of the aquatic biota by restricting the passage of sunlight. In this sense, the utilization of adsorbents, such as synthetic inorganic polymers (e.g., silica and zeolites), natural clays, and organic-inorganic hybrids (which allow for introduction of organic substances with interesting functional groups into inorganic supports) has been a noteworthy alternative. Another approach for the removal of azo-dyes from industrial effluents is their oxidative degradation by heterogeneous catalysts under mild conditions (room temperature and pressure, and use of environmentally friendly oxidants like hydrogen peroxide).

On the other hand, environmental problems concerning industrial oxidation reactions are mainly centered on the employed reagents. This area of fine chemistry is extremely important, because it is responsible for the production of various bulk chemicals, while it is the one field that most needs green innovations. One of the most promising alternatives in this area is the application of efficient/selective heterogeneous catalysts that can be employed in the presence of green oxidants like hydrogen peroxide.

Therefore, we propose to discuss these challenges and present some remarkable literature results reported by our research groups and others.

In: Chemistry Research Summaries Volume 12
Editor: Lucille Monaco Cacioppo

ISBN: 978-1-61668-757-1
© 2014 Nova Science Publishers, Inc.

Chapter 133

THE MITSUNOBU REACTION: FROM BENCH TO BATCH – CURRENT PERSPECTIVES AND FUTURE CHALLENGES

Brendan A. Burkett[*] and Paul B. Huleatt

Institute of Chemical and Engineering Sciences (ICES),
Agency for Science, Technology and Research (A[*]STAR),
Neuros, Singapore

RESEARCH SUMMARY

The Mitsunobu reaction involves the redox driven condensation of an acidic pro-nucleophile with primary and secondary alcohols. First reported in 1967, the classic version of this reaction involves activation of the alcohol with a reactive betaine intermediate derived from triphenylphosphine and diethylazodicarboxylate (DEAD) and substitution of the resulting triphenylphosphonium salt with the pro-nucleophile in an S_N2 fashion. Since the discovery of the Mitsunobu reaction, many variations have been reported to suit a wide range of synthetic applications on the bench scale, however several major drawbacks prevent widespread application in industry – most notably poor atom economy and waste generation. This chapter will review the current state of the art of the Mitsunobu reaction and discuss future challenges that lie in delivering sustainable variants for an industrial setting.

In: Chemistry Research Summaries Volume 12
Editor: Lucille Monaco Cacioppo

ISBN: 978-1-61668-757-1
© 2014 Nova Science Publishers, Inc.

Chapter 134

APPLICATION OF LACCASES IN ORGANIC SYNTHESIS: A REVIEW

*Kevin W. Wellington**

CSIR Biosciences, Enzyme Technologies Group,
Modderfontein, South Africa

RESEARCH SUMMARY

Laccases are oxidoreductases that are part of the family of multinuclear copper-containing oxidases. A feature of these enzymes is that they catalyze the monoelectronic oxidation of substrates using molecular oxygen and release water as the only by-product. Laccase substrates are typically phenols and amines, and the reaction products are dimers and oligomers derived from the coupling of reactive radical intermediates.

The search for new, efficient and environmentally benign processes for the textile and pulp and paper industries has increased interest in these 'green' catalysts. At present the application of laccases range from the textile to the pulp and paper industries and from food applications to bioremediation processes.

In recent years interest in the application of laccases in organic synthesis has grown with the development of Green Chemistry. This review provides an overview of the developments in the applications of laccases in primarily the field of organic synthesis. Other industrial applications such as that in the pulp and paper, textile, food and cosmetic industries will also be briefly discussed. It is anticipated that increased knowledge of the application of these enzymes will not only impact, but also revolutionize chemical, pharmaceutical and industrial processes.

---

* E-mail: kwellington@csir.co.za; kwwellington@gmail.com.

In: Chemistry Research Summaries Volume 12
Editor: Lucille Monaco Cacioppo

ISBN: 978-1-61668-757-1
© 2014 Nova Science Publishers, Inc.

Chapter 135

HYDROLASE-CATALYZED UNCONVENTIONAL REACTIONS AND APPLICATIONS IN ORGANIC SYNTHESIS

Na Wang and Xiao-Qi Yu *

Key Laboratory of Green Chemistry and Technology, Ministry of Education,
College of Chemistry, Sichuan University, Chengdu, P. R. China

RESEARCH SUMMARY

The potential of biocatalysis becomes increasingly recognized as an efficient and green tool for modern organic synthesis. Biocatalytic unconventional reactions, a new frontier extending the use of enzymes in organic synthesis, has attracted much attention and expanded rapidly in recent years. It focuses on the enzyme catalytic activities with unnatural substrates and alternative chemical transformations. Exploiting enzyme-catalytic unconventional reactions might lead to improvements in existing catalysts and provide novel synthesis pathways that are currently not available. Among these enzymes, hydrolase (such as lipase, protease, acylase) undoubtedly play an important role due to their high stability, wide sources and broad range of substrates. This chapter introduces the recent progress in hydrolase-catalytic unconventional reactions and application in organic synthesis. Some important examples of hydrolase catalytic unconventional reactions in addition reactions, oxidation reactions and polymerization reactions are reviewed.

---

* Fax: +86 28 85415886. E-mail: xqyu@scu.edu.cn.

In: Chemistry Research Summaries Volume 12   ISBN: 978-1-61668-757-1
Editor: Lucille Monaco Cacioppo   © 2014 Nova Science Publishers, Inc.

Chapter 136

BIOTECHNOLOGICAL ROUTES TO SYNTHESIZE PEPTIDE BASED HYDROGELS IN AQUEOUS MEDIUM

Cleofe Palocci and Laura Chronopoulou

Department of Chemistry, University of Rome "La Sapienza", Rome, Italy

RESEARCH SUMMARY

Peptide applications are growing significantly in the field of biomedicine (e.g., immunology, cell signaling, etc.). A recent projection valued that the global peptide therapeutics market would be worth nearly $2 billion in 2010. Such a significant and rapid development is due to the major clinical value that the specificity of peptides has been acknowledged. A growing number of applications in a wide range of treatments for such conditions as cancers, allergies, Parkinson's, multiple sclerosis, and heart failure is currently under development, with more than 400 peptide based drugs in advanced preclinical phases worldwide to this date. Among peptides, peptide based hydrogelators represent an extremely interesting class because they can trigger hydrogel formation giving rise to the formation of biocompatible biomaterials of biological relevance. For example, applications include tissue engineering and drug delivery systems. Moreover, self-assembling peptides could be used to develop injectable devices.

Recently, relevant research efforts are being made in the field of biofabrication of such self-assembling biomaterials. In particular, different classes of enzymes can be used to trigger the formation of peptidic bonds between precursors that form peptidic hydrogelators. Several enzymes derived from GRAS microorganisms can be employed to catalyze this reaction in aqueous medium, avoiding the use of organic solvents. Such novel, "green" synthetic procedures could have a strong impact on peptide production by introducing milder reaction conditions and limiting the use of harmful chemicals.

In: Chemistry Research Summaries Volume 12
Editor: Lucille Monaco Cacioppo

ISBN: 978-1-61668-757-1
© 2014 Nova Science Publishers, Inc.

Chapter 137

REDISCOVERING *CATHARANTHUS ROSEUS*: CHEMISTRY AND BIOLOGICAL ACTIVITY

David M. Pereira[1], Patrícia Valentão[1], Federico Ferreres[2], Mariana Sottomayor[3] and Paula B. Andrade[1]*

[1]REQUIMTE/Laboratório de Farmacognosia, Departamento de Química,
Faculdade de Farmácia, Universidade do Porto, R. Aníbal Cunha,
Porto, Portugal
[2]Research Group on Quality, Safety and Bioactivity of Plant Foods,
Department of Food Science and Technology, CEBAS (CSIC),
Espinardo (Murcia), Spain
[3]IBMC-Instituto de Biologia Molecular e Celular, Universidade
do Porto and Departamento de Botânica, Faculdade de Ciências,
Universidade do Porto, Porto, Portugal

ABSTRACT

Natural products remain today an important source of bioactive molecules to be used in human therapeutics. This interest arises mainly from the chemical diversity found in Nature and the ability of several organisms to synthesize a number of molecules whose complexity hinders their total or semi synthesis.

Catharanthus roseus (L.) G. Don (formerly *Vinca rosea* L.) is one of the most studied medicinal plants due to the accumulation in the leaves of the bisindole monoterpenic alkaloids vinblastine and vincristine, which were the first natural anticancer products to be clinically used. Together with a number of semisynthetic derivatives, these compounds are universally known as the Vinca alkaloids, which are still among the most valuable agents used in the treatment of cancer.

In the past few years, a number of studies focusing other biological properties of this species have emerged. In particular, the antioxidant activity and acetylcholinesterase inhibition of some of its primary and secondary metabolites have showed that, besides anticancer alkaloids, there might be an interest in exploiting this species for other medicinal activities and from a health-promoting point of view.

In this chapter, an update in *C. roseus* chemistry and bioactivity is presented. New metabolites and new pharmacological properties discovered in the last years using green chemistry approaches are reviewed, and the potential of further exploitation of *C. roseus* is discussed.